The Kent Ramblers Guide to the
Three River Valley
Walks in West Kent

Darent Valley Path
Eden Valley Walk
Medway Valley Walk

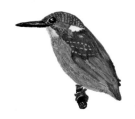

ISBN: 978-1-906494-76-6

Published by Kent Ramblers
www.kentramblers.org.uk

The Ramblers' Association is a registered charity in England & Wales (no: 1093577), a registered charity in Scotland (no: SC039799), and a company limited by guarantee registered in England and Wales (company registration no: 4458492).

Registered office: 2nd Floor, Camelford House, 87-90 Albert Embankment, London, SE1 7TW.

Front cover: Aylesford Old Bridge
Previous page: Kingfisher, associated with both Darent and Medway
This page: Gilridge near Penshurst

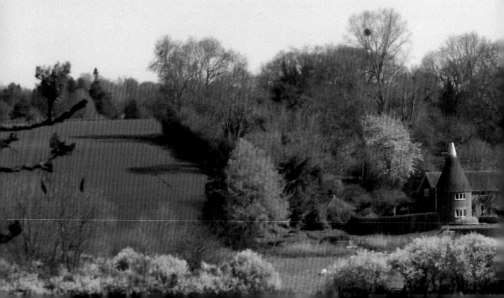

Contents

Disclaimer: Although we have made every effort to ensure that all information is accurate and up to date, we accept no responsibility for any loss, injury or inconvenience sustained by anyone using this guide. Please bear in mind that stiles are often removed or replaced by gates and paths are diverted for various reasons including riverbank erosion.

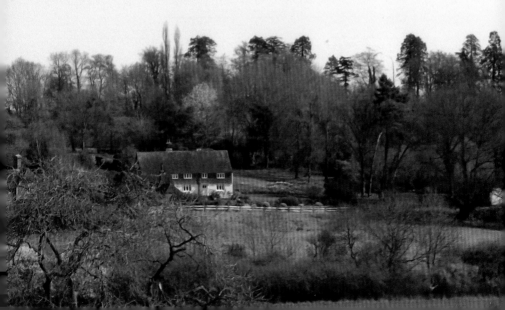

4

Introduction

Kent is traversed by a remarkable number of named walks. They are all attractive, they are all easily accessible by huge numbers of people in London, Surrey and Kent yet, in the main, they are not particularly well used. This is a huge shame and the purpose of this guide and others that we hope will follow is to remedy that. We do not expect to be so successful that the routes become busy, so exploring these walks is an opportunity to get away from the crowds and immerse yourself in Kent's landscape and history.

River valleys have long attracted both travellers and settlers. They have also been a source of power and a means of transport for finished goods, encouraging a variety of industries over the centuries. The Darent in particular has powered a huge concentration of watermills, first to grind corn and later to produce paper, all now gone or converted for other purposes. The Medway downstream from Maidstone has seen huge cement factories and brickworks come and go, leaving behind pits now water-filled to provide homes for wildlife and leisure activities for people. Along the Eden and the upper Medway the Wealden iron industry once thrived, leaving the many attractive furnace and hammer ponds that now enhance the landscape and the fine houses built by ironmasters with the profits from their trade.

The Medway valley was occupied in the iron age by a people who built megalithic tombs of which Kit's Coty House and Little Kit's Coty House are surviving examples. There were Roman villas every few miles along the Darent valley and the fine mosaics at Lullingstone Villa testify to the wealth of the inhabitants over several centuries. Aylesford claims to be the longest continually occupied village in Kent while Hever Castle in the Eden Valley and Penshurst Place near the confluence of the Eden and the the Medway are amongst the finest medieval houses in England and are rightly famous for their associations with major characters in English history.

Kent is of course known as "the garden of England". The hop gardens have largely gone while orchards, having declined markedly in the late 20th century, are seeing something of a revival albeit on a more intensive basis and with more of an eye to mechanisation than in the past. Soft fruit is being grown more and more under glass and in polytunnels, some of which you will pass along your way. Lavender growing has become popular in the Darent Valley,

Chiddingstone

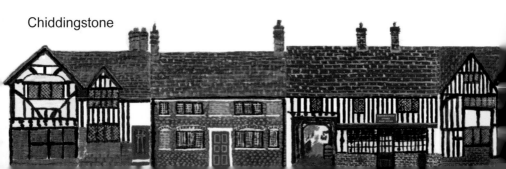

cereals and oil seed rape are common while along the Medway in particular are many meadows.

Inevitably in the busy county that is Kent, you will encounter the occasional unwelcome intrusion, particularly the motorways that carry traffic to and from the continent, but these are quickly passed and it is surprising how much tranquil countryside is to be found even in the more crowded parts of the county.

Walking these routes and researching the past and present of the surrounding landscape has been a pleasure and a revelation. If you want to understand and appreciate Kent, please follow in my footsteps.

Maps

The maps that follow have been carefully prepared to guide you on your way and at the time of publication are likely to be more up to date than available Ordnance Survey maps. That will change of course and in any case you may want maps that cover a wider area. For walking, Explorer maps (1:25,000) are far superior to Landranger maps (1:50,000). The Explorer maps that cover the three routes are:

Darent Valley Path: 147 (Sevenoaks & Tonbridge) and 162 (Greenwich & Gravesend)

Eden Valley Walk: 147 (Sevenoaks & Tonbridge)

Medway Valley Walk: 136 (High Weald) and 148 (Maidstone & The Medway Towns)

Planning and Equipment

These are not difficult walks. The main hazards are crossing roads and proximity to deep water, particularly at locks. The main planning issue is making your itinerary fit the times of buses and trains if required and the guide offers advice on doing this.

The only essential equipment is sturdy footwear and, in summer, sun cream and hat. And of course this guide. Many of the paths are very well made and suitable for walking shoes or even sturdy trainers. However, in wet weather there is always the risk of mud, with which boots will cope better. Boots give better foot and ankle support and in my opinion are to be preferred in all conditions but many people will disagree. Food, drink and a mobile phone are highly recommended on most sections, although you are rarely very far from a pub.

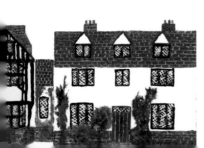
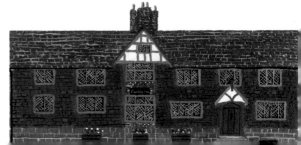

Evolution of the Landscape

Geology

The topography of Kent very much reflects the underlying geology, in particular the major rock formations dating from the Cretaceous period. These sandstones, clays and chalk were laid down in estuaries and shallow seas then uplifted during the Alpine earth movements to form what is known as the Wealden dome. Erosion sliced the top off the dome so that rock types that were originally laid down on top of each other are actually exposed as concentric rings with the oldest rocks (Tunbridge Wells sandstone) at the centre and the chalk of the North and South Downs at the edge (figure 1). The outer rings are cut by the coastline from the Seven Sisters west of Eastbourne to Thanet's North Foreland (figure 2), the harder elements forming exposed cliffs, and continue on the other side of the English Channel.

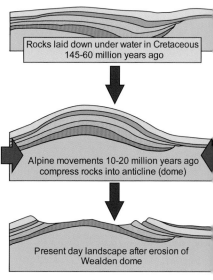

Figure 1

Inland the alternating bands of harder and softer layers result in a series of parallel ridges and valleys. In west Kent from north to south we have the North Downs chalk ridge, the Vale of Homesdale Gault clay valley, the Greensand ridge, the Vale of Kent Wealden clay valley and finally the dome of the Wealden sandstones (figure 3).

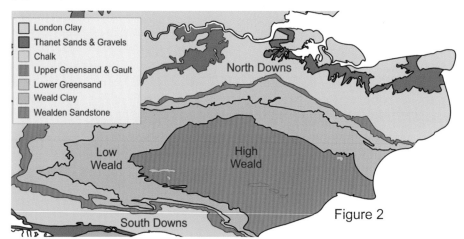

Figure 2

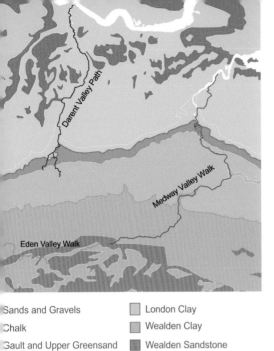

Sands and Gravels

Chalk

Gault and Upper Greensand

Lower Greensand

London Clay

Wealden Clay

Wealden Sandstone

Older Jurassic Rocks

Figure 3

Anomalous River System

It is a puzzle that the major rivers run not west to east along the valleys to discharge into the sea in east Kent but have cut their own valleys through the ridges northwards to the Thames (figure 4).

The Medway has its source near Turners Hill in the High Weald and flows initially north into the Low Weald. Here it follows the Vale of Kent eastwards past Tonbridge, then taking a northward cut through the Greensand ridge to Maidstone. Rather than flowing along the Vale of Holmesdale it continues northwards to cut through the North Downs and connect with the Thames north of Rochester.

The waters of the Darent begin their journey on the northerly slopes of the Greensand ridge and naturally flow into and then eastwards along the Vale of Holmesdale past the northern outskirts of Sevenoaks. Here the river turns sharply northwards and cuts a valley through the Downs through Shoreham to Farningham and then takes a natural course to Dartford and soon afterwards to the Thames.

The headwaters of the Eden lie in the Vale of Holmesdale no more than a couple of miles from the Darent yet they take a very different course to the Thames. Initially the Eden flows southward through the Greensand ridge before heading east through the clays of the Low Weald to join the Medway at Penshurst.

This pattern of drainage could not have developed under the current topography – rivers naturally flow along valleys and don't start cutting sideways through the higher ground that defines the valleys. These three

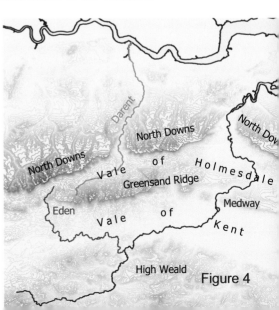

Figure 4

rivers are far from alone in southern England for being "discordant" with the current lie of the land and various theories have been advanced as to how this came about. One theory, that of "superimposition" is that the currently exposed rocks were once covered by a thick layer of some other material, perhaps clay, and that the river pattern was determined by the topography of that layer. As time went by the rivers cut their way through the clay, now largely gone, and then into the underlying rocks now exposed so that the river pattern that developed in the clay is superimposed on the present landscape.

An alternative theory is that the river pattern was established over the current strata before they were lifted and folded during the Alpine movements then eroded to create the ridges that would bar the establishment of such a pattern today. As the land rose, the rivers cut into the ridges along the already established routes faster than the land was uplifted so retaining their original courses.

There are other theories but for our purposes it is enough to note the curious routes taken by the rivers and the additional interest that results from passing through such a variety of landscape types.

Pill Boxes

Most walkers will have encountered pill boxes from time to time – usually brick or concrete structures, most of them relics of a huge national defence system from World War II. In the main they were placed alongside natural defensive features such as rivers and in particular the General Headquarters stop-line, which was planned to run across southern England then north to Edinburgh, incorporated both the Eden and Medway rivers. The map below indicates roughly the sites of those built and, although many have now been removed, you should spot quite a few on your journey.

The planned line was constructed as far north as Peterborough but then apparently there was a change of strategy and further construction abandoned.

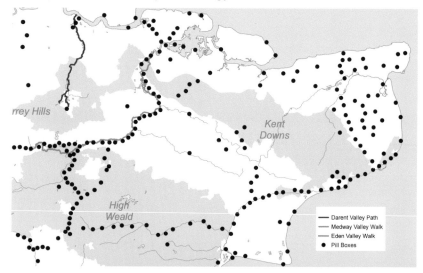

Wealden Hall Houses

Kent was a wealthy county in the middle ages and its more prosperous residents built some fine houses, many of which survive and can be seen along and around the three routes described in this book.

The most characteristic style in Tudor times was the hall house, an oak framed building whose defining feature was a large main room – the hall – open to the roof. There were typically four bays – the middle two formed the hall with an open fire and no chimney, hence the need to be open to the roof to allow the smoke to escape through the eaves. The bays at each end were normally split into two storeys with the upper storey being jettied out beyond the ground storey so that the hall was recessed behind the jetties.

The Wealden hall house, common in Kent and East Sussex but sometimes copied elsewhere, was characterised by a single hipped or half-hipped roof spanning all four bays whereas in other areas the two-storied sections were separately roofed.

The roof would originally have been thatched but most have subsequently been tiled. The oak frame is infilled with plaster and perhaps with upright studs that serve no structural function but are a status symbol whose number reflects the wealth of the owner.

Chimneys were later added to most hall houses, allowing a first floor to be built over the hall.

Many hall houses have been substantially altered. The plaster infill may have been replaced with brick or the upper storey may have been hung with tiles. Sometimes the evidence of a building's history may only be visible internally but very often there are at least a few clues to be spotted as you pass by.

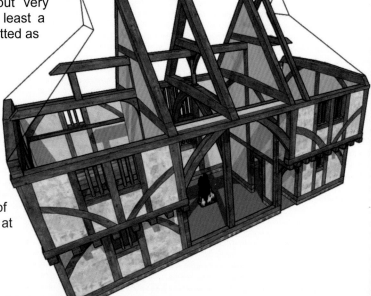

Typical Wealden Hall House – note the half-hipped roof (with small gables at the top) and the jettied end bays

Darent Valley Path

The section of the Darent Valley from Otford to Farningham falls within the Kent Downs Area of Outstanding Natural Beauty. The picturesque qualities of the area were made famous by the "Valley of Vision" landscape paintings of Samuel Palmer who lived in Shoreham from 1826 to 1835. The rest of the valley may be less picturesque but much of it is surprisingly rural and all of it is full of history.

The origin of the name Darent (alternatively Darenth) is variously explained but the most popular interpretation is that the name is derived from early English words meaning "river of oaks".

The valley has been a welcoming environment for man for as long as there have been people in Britain. Fertile soils, a route of communication and transport and later a source of power have all been exploited over the centuries. Stone Age flints, Bronze Age axe heads, Roman villas, Saxon cemeteries, Norman churches, Medieval hall houses, a Tudor palace, water mills aplenty and gunpowder and explosives factories make a far from complete list of artefacts evidencing the vibrant life of the valley. There is much to see along the way.

The path has alternative starting points at Chipstead and at Sevenoaks station. There is a car park (and a pub) at the former but the latter is very convenient for those wishing to return to their starting point by train as the line from Bromley to Sevenoaks passes through Eynsford, Shoreham and Otford. The routes merge at the railway bridge immediately before the lavender fields just south of Otford.

At the time of writing there is talk of extending the route to start from Westerham and so achieve more complete coverage of the Darent Valley. If this welcome development comes about it is likely to be several years hence.

Few parts of the described walking route are available to cyclists but the valley is well provided with roads and lanes apart from the last section across the marshes. However, the section from Powder Mill Lane at Brooklands past Brooklands Lake and through Dartford Park then through Dartford town to the railway station is an attractive traffic-free route (Sustrans route 125).

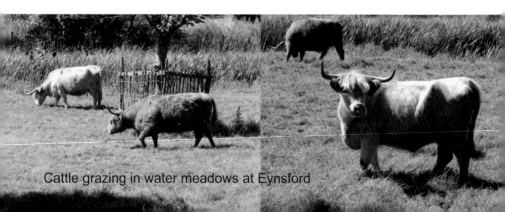

Cattle grazing in water meadows at Eynsford

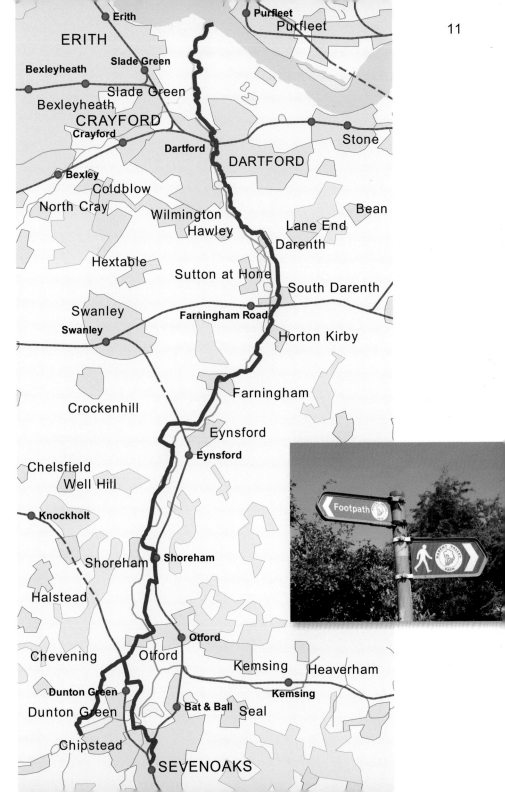

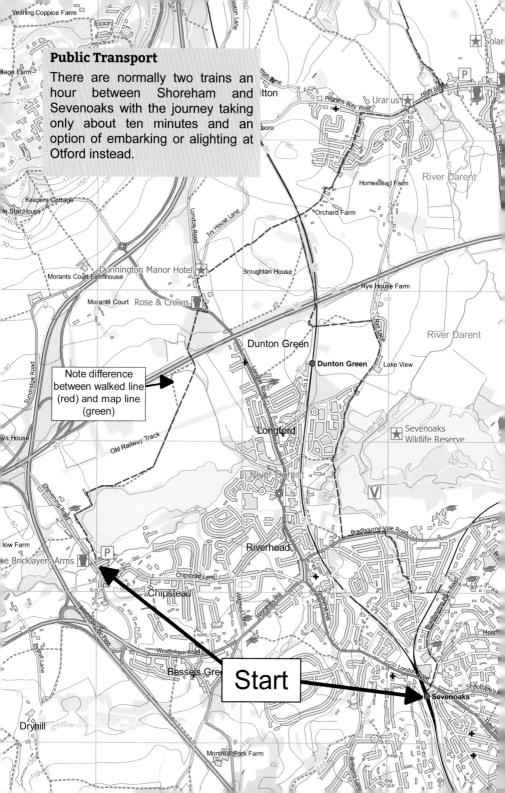

Public Transport

There are normally two trains an hour between Shoreham and Sevenoaks with the journey taking only about ten minutes and an option of embarking or alighting at Otford instead.

Note difference between walked line (red) and map line (green)

Start

Sevenoaks or Chipstead to Shoreham (5.4 miles)

There are two starting points for the DVP. For those travelling by train there is a route starting at Sevenoaks station. Alternatively there is a route starting at a car park at the western end of a flooded gravel pit at Chipstead. The two routes join at the bridge over the railway line just before Orchard Farm on the outskirts of Otford.

Sevenoaks Station to Orchard Farm

Emerging from the station, turn right along main road to pedestrian crossing, cross, turn left and then right into Hitchen Hatch Lane. Take first turn on left – Bradbourne Park Road – and go downhill to lowest point, then as you start climbing again look for unmade Clock House Lane on left. Take lane uphill over railway and down again to Lambarde Road. Turn right and soon go through gate on left into Bradbourne Lakes Park. Keep right through the park past the wildfowl ponds to Betenson Avenue. Go straight across into the northern part of park, keeping right past pond and emerging on Bradbourne Vale Road. Cross and turn left until at the end of the pasture on the right there is a rough track. Go through gate just a few metres up the track and walk across grass directly away from the road towards woodland.

Follow path through woodland with Sevenoaks Wildlife Reserve on your right then along track to Rye Lane. Turn right and follow lane, soon curving gently left. Opposite entrance to Wickens Meadow Residential Park take path over stile on left. Head directly away from road (at an angle of about ten degrees left of the fence) to the trees on the railway embankment at the far side of the field where there is a tunnel under the railway. Through the tunnel the path officially bears half right then half right again to a gap in the fence but a more obvious path going immediately sharp right will get you to the same place. Turn right along a track under the M26 then bear right up bank and keep close to railway line to top of hill. Take first bridge over railway bridge on right and down track past Orchard Farm.

Chipstead to Orchard Farm

From close to the car park entrance, cross grassy area past information board and take path between hedge and fence with lake on right. Cross bridge over stream (Darent) entering the lake and continue along backs of gardens and school grounds. At corner go right and at next corner left then emerge to cross grassy area diagonally to kissing gate. Soon after reaching open meadow, cross track and field to hedge then bear left diagonally through gap in hedge along old railway track. Continue in same direction to corner of field and track leading to underpass beneath M26. On the other side climb up bank, bear right through gate, up steps and in straight line through newly-planted woodland to road at Dunton Green.

Turn right to road junction then left along London Road and take path on right just before the Donnington Manor Hotel (North Downs Way, signposted "Otford"). Follow path between fence and hedge then uphill along right hand

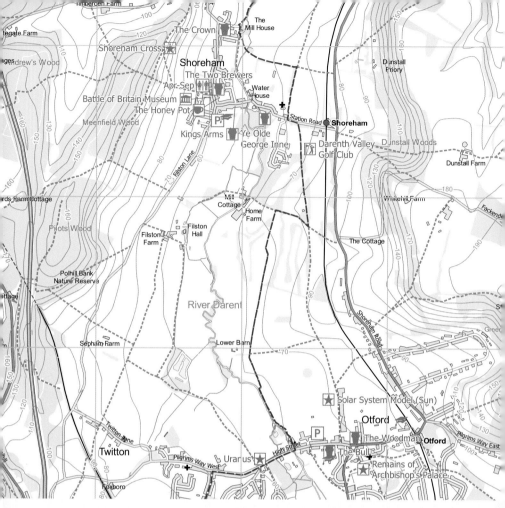

edge of field. Through short section of woodland, cross field to bridge over railway to Orchard Farm.

Orchard Farm to Shoreham

From railway bridge, follow asphalt track, to outskirts of Otford. There used to be fine lavender fields here but lately they have looked neglected and may soon be gone. Continue in same direction along road to meet Pilgrim's Way at T junction. Turn right downhill, cross bridge over the Darent and 100 or so metres further on take path on left along drive with mill race

on your left towards house straddling the race. (To visit Otford's various facilities, keep straight on up the High Street and return to this point.)

Keep to right of house and out into field. Follow path parallel to left hand edge of field to gate. Continue across next field to junction of paths. Take path through gate just left of straight ahead. Follow top of field then enter woodland. Continue to lane.

Turn right uphill. Soon after passing entrance to cricket pavilion on left, take path on left between fences. Skirt edge of cricket field and resume path between fences. Continue to Station Road. Turn left and take path on right just before wall starts.

After a few metres there is gate on the left into the churchyard. If you want to explore Shoreham, go through churchyard into village. For the next section of the DVP, carry straight on.

Points of Interest between Sevenoaks/Chipstead and Shoreham

Sevenoaks Wildlife Reserve

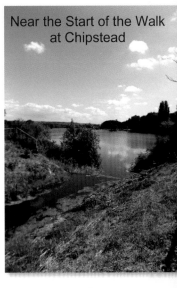

Near the Start of the Walk at Chipstead

These flooded gravel pits set in woodland are operated by Kent Wildlife Trust and are free to visit any day. There is a visitor centre with café and toilets but it is not open every day (usually Wednesday to Sunday). It is possible to walk all the way round the second largest lake. The paths on the north and south sides of the largest lake are dead ends at present so you must retrace your steps but there are welcome plans to extend them all the way round. There are several hides on the south side from which to view the wildfowl. At the time of writing plans have just been announced for a visually striking new visitor centre to replace the current building which has seen better days.

Solar System Model

As you walk along Pilgrims Way West towards Otford High Street you will pass a concrete pillar labelled "Uranus" on the other side of the road on your left. This is part of a scale model of the solar system with pillars to represent the sun and all of the planets. The pillars for the sun and the nearer planets are in the recreation ground off the high street. The model, the largest in the world, was created to celebrate the millennium and shows the relative positions of the Sun and planets at midnight on 1 January 2000. Considerable effort was required to design an accurate layout that gave public access to every planet.

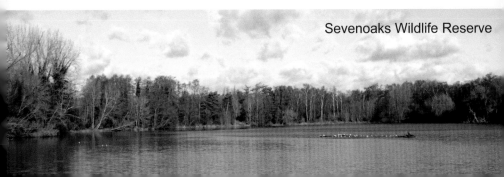

Sevenoaks Wildlife Reserve

On the same scale, the nearest star would be in Los Angeles!

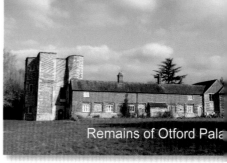
Remains of Otford Palace

Otford

The village is worth a detour. There are many listed buildings on or around the High Street, most famously the duck pond in the middle of the roundabout opposite the church.

The first house on your right as you enter the village, largely hidden from view behind tall fences, is Broughton Manor. For nearly three centuries until 1830 a house on this site was the home of the Polhill family whose estate included much land around Otford and Shoreham. Monuments to various members of the family adorn Otford church. The steep road carrying the A224 up the North Downs is known as Polhill (the name being taken by the nearby garden centre and Kent Wildlife Trust nature reserve) and, as the family name predates their move from Detling in 1554, the "hill" must be named from the family rather than vice versa.

Battles of Otford

It is recorded in the Anglo Saxon Chronicle that in 776AD the forces of Offa, King of Mercia, fought those of Kent at Otford. Sources have differing views as to who won. Kent was eventually absorbed into Mercia but the outcome may have been delayed by the battle.

There was a clearer outcome to a battle here in 1016 when Edmund Ironside defeated Canute and the Danes.

Polhill Bank

Home to many common chalk grassland flowers, this reserve run by Kent Wildlife Trust can be visited along public footpaths from Otford and Shoreham or by parking in the lay-by at the top of Polhill. At the time of writing an appeal is under way for funding to add substantially to the area of the reserve.

Otford Archbishop's Palace

The construction of Otford Palace was begun in 1514 by William Warham, Archbishop of Canterbury. The following year Cardinal Wolsey began the building of Hampton Court. The similarity of layout and architectural style of the two buildings suggests that the two men were expressing their political rivalry in competition to build the finest palace. Otford

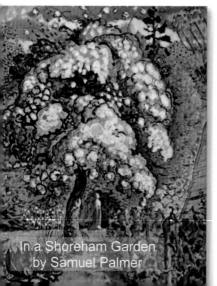
In a Shoreham Garden by Samuel Palmer

emerged as the larger building and was subsequently transferred to Henry VIII in an exchange of lands by Warham's successor, Thomas Cranmer. After Henry's death the palace was neglected and fell into decay as it was gradually plundered by local landowners as a source of building materials. The most prominent remnant, the north west tower, can still be visited.

Sepham Farm

The three oast houses enhance the view from the hills but from the DVP you may only glimpse their bright white cowls. The farmhouse is a late medieval hall house. Kent County Council's original guide to the DVP says that the name derives from Anglo-Saxon for "settlement on swampy ground" but Historic England claim that it comes from John de Cepham who owned the manor in the reign of Henry III – take your choice.

Filston Hall

Another very fine building with parts dating back to the sixteenth century and perhaps earlier, surrounded by a medieval moat. There are four fine white-cowled oast houses. Around 1528 Thomas Cromwell of *Wolf Hall* fame (Hilary Mantel's book and the BBC TV adaptation) took out a lease on the manor but was apparently acting as middleman for a Robert Studley and never occupied the property. The hall lies on the original line of the Darent; its present course is the result of a diversion to help irrigate the surrounding fields and supply an adequate head of water to the corn mill.

Shoreham Corn Mill

The corn mill was situated south of the village where Mill Cottage now stands. There is nothing to be seen of the original mill.

Samuel Palmer

Water House is known as the home of artist Samuel Palmer who lived in Shoreham from 1826 to 1835. Initially he lived in a run-down cottage nicknamed "Rat Abbey" but when his father, Samuel senior, rented half of what was then called "Waterhouse" in 1828 Samuel junior moved in with him. Palmer was much influenced by William Blake to pursue a mystical interpretation of landscape and it was during his time at Shoreham that this was expressed most strongly.

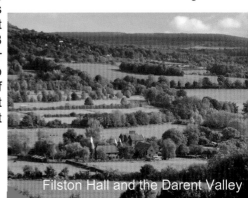
Filston Hall and the Darent Valley

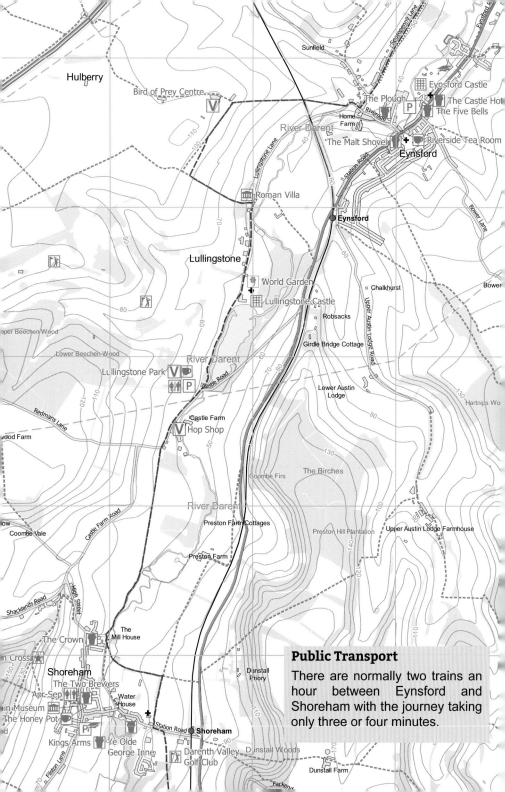

Public Transport

There are normally two trains an hour between Eynsford and Shoreham with the journey taking only three or four minutes.

Shoreham to Eynsford (3.8 miles)

From the gate at the top of Shoreham churchyard turn left in a northerly direction along left hand edge of field. When the hedge ends on the left, turn left downhill, initially following the hedge on the left and then curving right to meet the Darent near a footbridge.

(Alternatively go through the churchyard and into Church Street past Ye Olde George Inne. Go downhill to the river and turn left before the stone bridge, passing to the left of Water House, and continue along the riverbank to the footbridge.)

Across the bridge, turn right to join Mill Lane and bear right to take path on left, soon following the river bank. After passing through a couple of gates, climb gently away from the river along broad track between fences then bear left across open field. At a gate cross concrete track and cross field towards gate in long row of trees. Continue in same direction to Redmans Lane.

Bear left across lane and up bank to take permissive path along bottom of lavender field with Castle Farm and Hop Shop on right. On reaching junction of lanes cross to enter the grounds of the Lullingstone Park

Visitor Centre (or just take path between Centre and river if not visiting the Centre).

Go past the building and turn right through gate to join riverside path, keeping river on your right. Continue past Lullingstone Castle and World Garden on right and along lane to Lullingstone Roman Villa.

You have a choice here. The official path goes up steps just before the villa and the route to Eynsford via the Eagle Heights Bird of Prey Centre offers fine views of the valley allowing you to look down on the viaduct. However, the route can be very muddy when wet and you have the alternative of just following the lane along the valley under the viaduct.

If taking the official route, follow path up the steps, climbing along left hand edge of field to first hedge on right. Turn right along lower side of hedge to drive leading to Eagle Heights Bird of Prey Centre. Cross drive and bear right across field to railway crossing. Cross carefully and descend to lane. Turn left and follow road round to right.

At first junction you may wish to go straight on to visit the picturesque ford, church, castle and places of refreshment at Eynsford but to continue along the DVP to Farningham turn left along Sparepenny Lane.

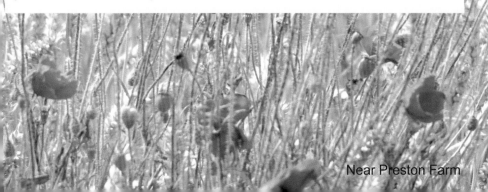

Near Preston Farm

Points of Interest between Shoreham and Eynsford

Shoreham Cross

On the hillside and easily accessible by public footpaths (although a bit of a climb from the village), this memorial to the fallen of the First World War is made of compacted chalk and was completed in 1921.

Shoreham Aircraft Museum

As befits its location not too far from Biggin Hill and in the most bombed village in England during World War II, the museum focuses on artefacts from the Battle of Britain. There is a tea room and garden. Normally open Saturdays, Sundays and bank holidays from Easter to Remembrance Sunday.

The Mill House

The Domesday book of 1086 records a corn mill on or near the site but in the 1690s it was converted by French Huguenots into a paper mill and remained in operation until 1926. The remains of a Roman bath house have been discovered nearby.

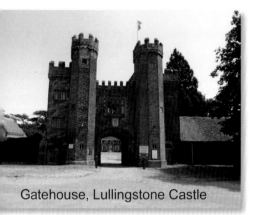
Gatehouse, Lullingstone Castle

Castle Farm and the Hop Shop

Castle Farm is a mixed farm producing beef and vegetables but most conspicuously the lavender and hops seen in the surrounding fields and for sale in the shop.

Lullingstone Country Park

Operated by Kent County Council, the visitor centre has a car park, toilets and a popular cafe. The park was once a deer park and the remains of the high iron deer fence that once surrounded it can still be seen in places. The park is now shared between a golf course and the country park with its woodland and wildflower meadows.

Lullingstone Castle

The red brick gatehouse dates from 1492, although the right hand tower has been restored after being hit by a flying bomb in 1944. The main manor house has a Queen Anne west facade which houses the main entrance but there are surviving parts of the original Tudor building to the north and east facades. It was not called

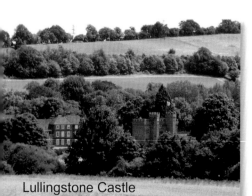
Lullingstone Castle

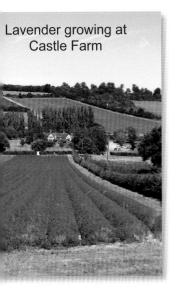

Lavender growing at Castle Farm

a "castle" until the middle of the 18th century. Normally open Fridays, Saturdays, Sundays and Bank Holiday Mondays in the summer season.

In 1932 a silk farm with mulberry trees was established here by the then Lady Hart Dyke. Silk from the farm was used for both Queen Elizabeth's wedding dress and coronation robes. The business was sold and moved elsewhere in the 1950s. For many visitors the most memorable feature of the wormery was its awful smell.

Within the walled garden, a "World Garden of Plants" has been created. There is a (somewhat distorted) world map with each country represented by its native plants. The new garden opened in 2005. The project was the subject of a BBC TV series broadcast in 2006 & 2007 narrating the not inconsiderable difficulties encountered by the Hart Dyke family who own the house but struggle to pay the bills. Whether the walled garden is large enough to do real justice to the concept you will have to judge for yourself should you visit.

Lullingstone Roman Villa

Managed by English Heritage, this important site with its exceptional mosaics, clear ground plan and the earliest recorded place of Christian worship in Britain is well worth a visit. The remains are covered with a recently renewed building that contains impressive displays of Roman artefacts. Occupied from around AD 100 to AD 400, the villa was excavated in the 1950s.

Eagle Heights Bird of Prey Centre

The centre accommodates a wide variety of birds of prey with demonstrations twice daily when open (daily in summer and weekends in winter). There are also mammals including huskies and some reptiles.

Eynsford Viaduct

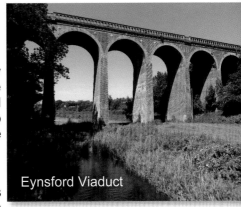

Eynsford Viaduct

The viaduct with its nine brick arches topped with a stone balustrade was opened in 1862 and still carries the railway from London to Sevenoaks (via Bat and Ball, not the more direct route via Orpington), Maidstone and beyond.

Eynsford to South Darenth (3.2 miles)

From the road junction near Home Farm follow Sparepenny Lane all the way to Farningham. There is currently an option of walking on a permissive path in the field adjacent to Sparepenny Lane on the right – there have been various such arrangements under the government's Environmental Stewardship Scheme and its predecessors but there is no guarantee that one will be in place at the time of your visit. Turn right at T-junction downhill to bridge over the Darent.

Leave the High Street through the garden of the Lion Hotel along a path close to the river. Approaching the A20, cross the Darent by wooden footbridge then turn sharp left under A20. Continue with river on your left under M20. Follow river as it bears right then bear left along path between river and fence, soon turning right away from river then left across fields to Franks Lane.

Turn left, don't take first path on right but cross the bridge over the Darent and take path immediately on right along the wooded river bank. At end of wood when river bears right, go straight ahead along field edge then diagonally across next field to recreation ground. Keep to right hand edge of recreation ground and take path between river on right and lakes on left, emerging on Station Road at South Darenth.

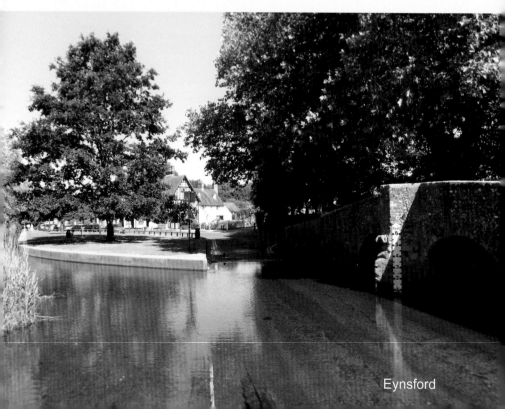

Eynsford

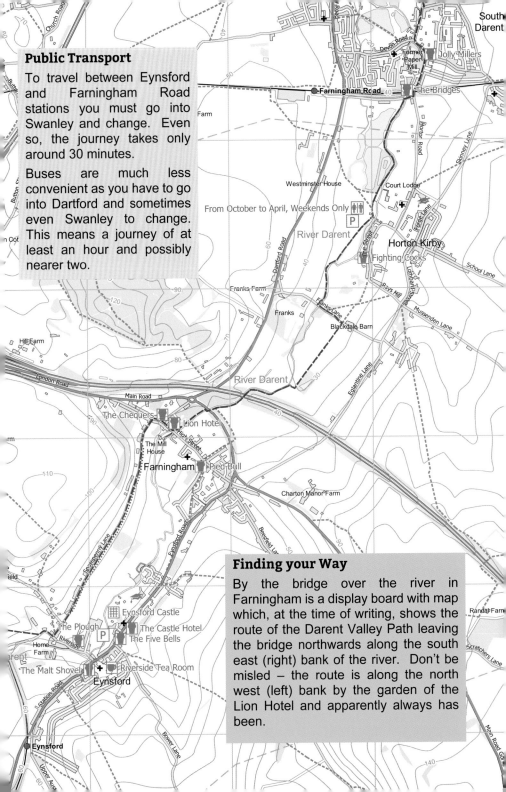

Public Transport

To travel between Eynsford and Farningham Road stations you must go into Swanley and change. Even so, the journey takes only around 30 minutes.

Buses are much less convenient as you have to go into Dartford and sometimes even Swanley to change. This means a journey of at least an hour and possibly nearer two.

Finding your Way

By the bridge over the river in Farningham is a display board with map which, at the time of writing, shows the route of the Darent Valley Path leaving the bridge northwards along the south east (right) bank of the river. Don't be misled – the route is along the north west (left) bank by the garden of the Lion Hotel and apparently always has been.

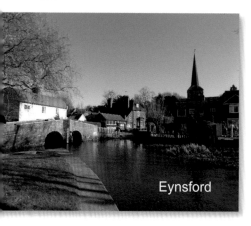
Eynsford

Points of Interest between Eynsford and South Darenth

Eynsford Village

The ford and hump back bridge over the Darent, with either the Norman church or the Tudor cottage in the background depending which way you are looking, is a greatly photographed and painted scene that testifies to the antiquity of the village. Scattered amongst the more modern houses strung along the main road you will still find a good number of worthy old buildings.

Eynsford Castle

This small Norman castle was held in the twelfth century by William de Eynsford who fell out with Archbishop Thomas Becket by whom he was then excommunicated. After Becket's death in 1170 the strength of public feeling against his enemies forced William to abandon the castle never to return. Or so the story goes. More reliable sources indicate that the castle was not abandoned until 1312 following a dispute over inheritance of the castle after the de Eynsford family died out. The building consists of the remains of a hall surrounded by a high curtain wall, both made predominantly of flints.

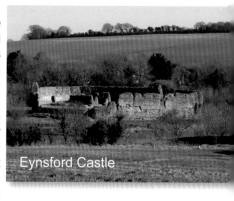
Eynsford Castle

Sparepenny Lane

So named because you could spare ("save") a penny by using it rather than the main road which carried a toll. There are many similarly named roads across the country.

Farningham

In the eighteenth and early nineteenth centuries the village was a major overnight stop for those travelling by coach between London and the Kent coast. Most of the fine surviving buildings are from that era when there were many coaching inns catering for different

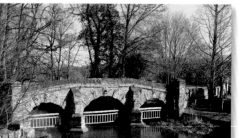
Farningham cattle screen?

sections of society. The Lion Hotel catered for the grandest clientele including officers and gentry while the Bull Inn was more popular with farmers and tradesmen.

Cattle Screen

The purpose of this structure, pictured, is not known with certainty but the prevailing hypothesis is that it was to prevent cattle from wandering downstream while crossing the ford. It seems rather more ornate than necessary for the job it did and was presumably intended to show off the landowner's wealth.

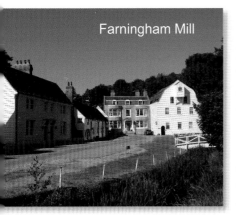
Farningham Mill

Farningham Mill

The mill and associated buildings make a charming ensemble. There has been a mill here at least since the Domesday book and probably much longer. The present white weather-boarded mill and brick house were built in the eighteenth century by Charles Colyer whose family continued to own the property until 2010 despite the grinding of corn ceasing in 1900 or thereabouts. Not all the buildings you see are old – in particular the second building on the left was built since 2012 as part of a project to convert all buildings into residential units.

Franks

The name derives from the Frankish family who owned the estate from the thirteenth to the fifteenth century. The surviving house was built in 1591 by Lancelot Bathurst and reputedly Elizabeth I stayed there. During the Second World Way the house was a maternity hospital and in recent decades it has been used as the headquarters of various companies. At the time of writing the front of the house has been behind scaffolding for several months while building work takes place.

Church of St Mary the Virgin, Horton Kirby

The original Norman church was built around 1220 (views vary) by masons from the team working on Rochester Cathedral. A new nave was built following an earthquake in 1382, somewhat offset to the south from the original line of symmetry, and the original steeple was replaced with a brick tower in 1817.

South Darenth to Dartford (4.2 miles)

If coming from Farningham Road railway station, turn left downhill parallel to the railway, cross the main road, continue downhill to cross the Darent then turn left under the viaduct.

If continuing from previous section of path, turn right over Darent to T-junction then left under railway viaduct.

Pass former paper mill, now converted to residential accommodation but retaining its landmark chimney. At The Jolly Millers pub bear left but keep right at next junction along lane with the Darent, or at least one branch of it, on your left. Just around a corner as lane begins to climb, take path along track on left. Soon leave track on path on right alongside fence. Go straight across field to small parking area then take the leftmost path ahead close to the river bank. When forced to do so, bear right out of wood and along bottom edge of field; on approaching industrial site bear left down steps and along path between fences to Darenth Hill.

Bear right to lane opposite (Darenth Road) and follow past The Chequers pub until you reach the entrance to the Beechcare Care Home. Just a few metres further on, take path on left across field to meet river at corner. Bear right along track under the M25 and along bank of Darent to bridge. Over the bridge, turn right then left along track to main road at Hawley.

Turn right and shortly after passing under the A2 take track on right directly away from the road towards the Darent. On reaching the river at a bridge, don't cross but turn left along bank following well-made track to next bridge. Cross the river then bear left along the opposite bank with the river on your left. On reaching lane at Brooklands, turn left across Darent and almost immediately turn right across parking area to gap in metal fence. Go straight forward between lake on left and Darent on right. As you approach the A225 (Princes Road) embankment, bear right under road. (Should the tunnel under the road be closed, instead take next path on left which climbs the embankment and cross the A225 very carefully. Turn right and soon take path on left which zigzags down the embankment.)

Bear right directly away from the road past athletics track (with Darent on the right) and pass skating park inside fenced area on left. Bear left here to centre of park then turn right past bandstand and along central path through park to street by library. Bear left to pedestrian crossing and cross end of bus station to Market Place; continue forward to pedestrianised High Street. Turn right, pass to right of church then sharp left along riverside path. There are waymarks in the surface of High Street – see inside back cover.

Follow path under main road and continue along riverside to the last footbridge before the railway on the embankment ahead. For Dartford railway station, turn left here. For the next section of the DVP, continue along riverside path through tunnel under railway.

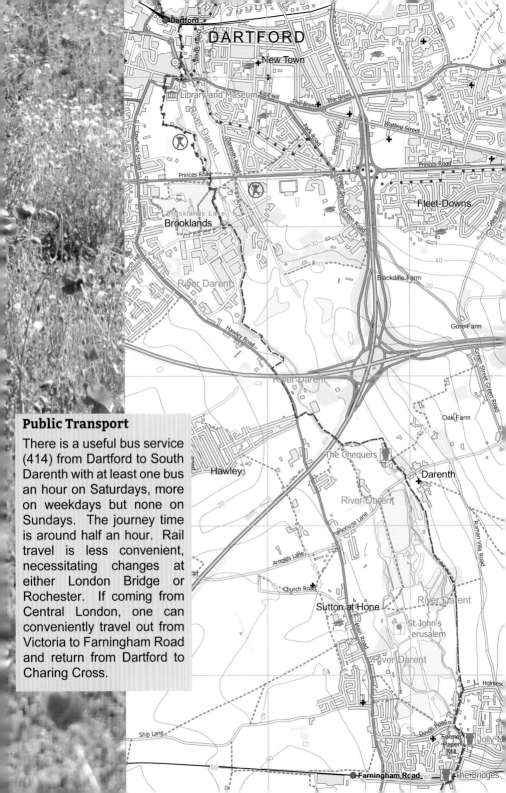

Public Transport

There is a useful bus service (414) from Dartford to South Darenth with at least one bus an hour on Saturdays, more on weekdays but none on Sundays. The journey time is around half an hour. Rail travel is less convenient, necessitating changes at either London Bridge or Rochester. If coming from Central London, one can conveniently travel out from Victoria to Farningham Road and return from Dartford to Charing Cross.

Places of Interest between South Darenth and Dartford

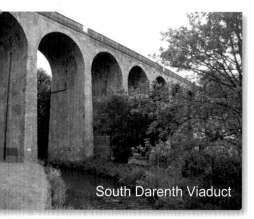
South Darenth Viaduct

South Darenth Viaduct

The brick viaduct, consisting of 10 arches each 10 metres wide and 20 metres above the river. was built in 1859-60 to carry the London, Chatham and Dover Railway over the valley.

South Darenth Paper Mill

Authorities differ as to whether this mill, also known as Horton Kirby paper mill, was ever water-powered. Certainly it was powered by steam turbines in its heyday. The inventors of the world's first continuous papermaking machine installed one here in the early 1800s. The mill was hugely successful and by the 1950s was employing 450 people. Thereafter the business declined steadily, paper making ceased in 2003 and much of the site has now been converted into residential units. Manufacture of wood chip wallpaper continued until early 2018.

The surviving chimney, one of two, is dated 1881. In 1918 a 70 ft circular extension was added (although the BBC's Domesday project recorded that the extension was only 35 ft and added in 1914). The extension was reduced by half in the late twentieth century and now none of it remains.

Pape
Mill

The Jolly Millers

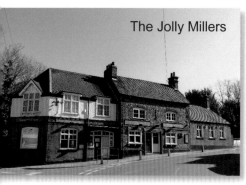
The Jolly Millers

According to the pub's former landlord, the central part of the building, now faced with flint and edged in brick, dates to 1540 and was once a charnel house. The extensions to each side were added much later.

St John's Jerusalem Garden

Belonging to the National Trust, only the moated garden and the remains of a 13th century chapel built by the Knights Hospitaller are open to the public, normally on Wednesday afternoons in the summer months. The fine house was largely built by Abraham Hill who acquired the property in 1665 and created the orchard of apple and pear trees. The Kent historian Edward Hasted owned

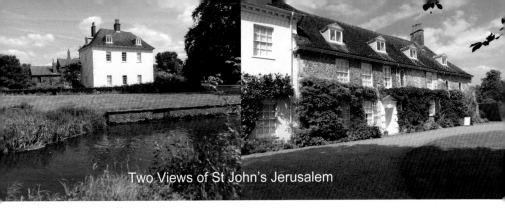
Two Views of St John's Jerusalem

the house from 1755-76 and spent so much money on it that he became bankrupt and was imprisoned for six years. Hasted's great work *"The History and Topographical Survey of the County of Kent"* was written here.

Brooklands Lakes

The site was part of a gunpowder factory from 1732 to 1906 (the rest of the fifty acre factory was on the other side of Powder Mill Lane and on the other side of the Darent). There were many explosions and fatalities over the years. Gravel extraction created huge pits that then filled with water to form the lakes that now provide a haven for ducks, geese and fishermen.

Dartford

Dartford is an ancient town situated where the Roman road of Watling Street, the remains of which are beneath the High Street, crossed the Darent. The church of the Holy Trinity is generally reckoned to be worth a visit and amongst the town's other claims to fame are as the place where Richard Trevithic (engineer of the industrial revolution) died in poverty in 1833 and where Mick Jagger met Keith Richards in 1961, an encounter which led to the formation of the Rolling Stones pop group. Anne of Cleves was given the Manor House by Henry VIII on dissolution of their marriage but only the gatehouse remains, in a fenced off area adjacent to the B&Q car park, now used for wedding ceremonies.

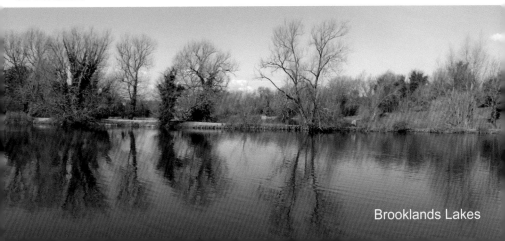
Brooklands Lakes

Dartford to the Thames (2.1 miles – but you will have to walk back too)

Emerging from Dartford station, turn left to rear of building then turn right downhill with railway line immediately on your left. At bend take path on left towards footbridge over Darent but descend steps before crossing the river and double back under footbridge and railway. Turn left up Mill Pond Lane to roundabout. Go anticlockwise round roundabout and turn right into Hythe Street passing the Hufflers Arms. Take path on right between fences, cross Darent and turn left into corner of car park. Take path along riverside and stick as closely as you can to the bank – ignore any signs that appear to direct you away from the river.

Soon after passing under a gantry you will pass the remains of the derelict lock (see Points of Interest); keep going towards University Way and take the path underneath. Now follow the flood embankment which meanders towards the flood barrier at the mouth of the Darent. Although there are various paths shown on the map, the only obvious route on the ground is the Darent Valley Path so you shouldn't go far wrong. If visibility is good you will be able to see your destination, the Dartford Creek flood barrier, although its apparent direction will constantly change as your route weaves back and forth along the embankment. Pass the barrier and follow the bank to the right to finish at a metal tower,

described on large scale maps as a navigation light. There is nothing else here to signify that you have reached your destination. Until 1957 there was a pub here, the Long Reach Tavern, but it was demolished when the sea defences were built, so if you want a celebratory drink you will have to bring it with you.

Points of Interest between Dartford and the Thames

Dartford and Crayford Navigation

The Darent and Cray used to be busy waterways with barges bringing wheat to local mills. The confluence of the two rivers is about a mile upstream from the Thames and just over half a mile further up the Darent branch there are the derelict remains of a lock that used to allow barges to continue upriver to Dartford. The Dartford and Crayford Creek Trust was established in 2016 to improve the navigation and you may see signs of their work as you pass the lock.

Joyce Green

The marshy area on your right as you approach the Thames was once the site of the Joyce Green Aerodrome. Already in use by Vickers, after the outbreak of World War I it was taken over by the Royal Flying Corps for pilot training. The RFC having moved to Biggin Hill in 1917, the Joyce Green Aerodrome was returned to agricultural use soon after

ains and buses will get you to ur starting point but will not turn you from your destination you will have to walk back.

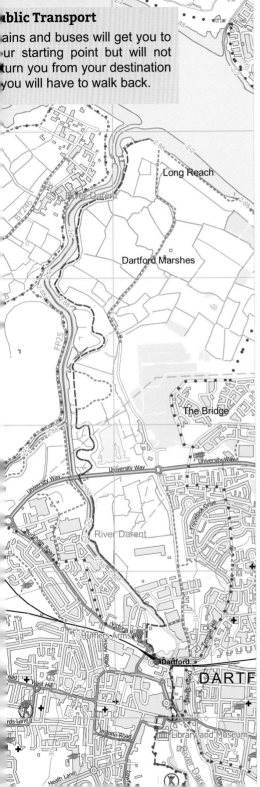

the war ended and the buildings were all dismantled by 1940.

The area was also for many years home to a fireworks factory. The fireworks were made and stored in small, well-separated huts so that an explosion in one would not start a chain reaction in the others. In 1953 the area flooded and the reaction of water with chemicals stored on the site caused an explosion that shattered 500 panes of glass in the windows of the nearby Joyce Green Hospital which closed in 2000. For much of the first half of the twentieth century there were three isolation hospitals on Dartford Marshes, two of them identified on old maps as being for sufferers from smallpox.

The name comes from a thirteenth century landowner called Joceus de Marisco.

Flood Barrier

The large structure at the mouth of the Darent allows gates to be lowered to prevent an exceptionally high tide on the Thames from inundating the land.

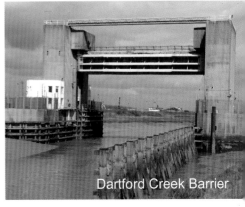

Dartford Creek Barrier

The Wealden Iron Industry

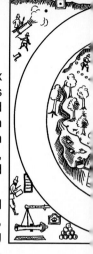

Many of what are now the most rural parts of Kent and Sussex were once amongst the most industrialised parts of Britain thanks to the iron industry that thrived here firstly in Roman times and even more strongly in the Tudor and Stuart periods. Although the industry has entirely gone now and was largely based on an area south of that traversed by the walks described in this book, the wealth generated by the second phase of the industry funded many of the fine houses in the area.

In the Tudor and Stuart periods the hills and ghylls of the Weald were alive with the mining of iron ore, the burning of charcoal, the smelting of iron in bloomeries and furnaces and the working of iron in forges using huge hammers driven by water power. The noise, the smoke, the felling of trees, the traffic transporting the raw materials and finished products and the heaps of industrial waste would have horrified the conservationists of the time, had there been any – and in fact there were a few protesting at the large scale of woodland clearance. Ironically, today we value many of the features of the landscape created by this industry.

Some a
taken in
local ir
Wea

The Weald is made up of sandstones and clays that formed in shallow inland waters and became rich in iron. The many references on OS maps to chalybeate springs (iron-rich waters thought by some to have health-giving properties) are evidence of this and the red sludge sometimes seen in Wealden ghylls is due to the iron content. The Weald is also rich in timber, the other raw material necessary for primitive iron production. These factors, together with proximity to its customer base, especially the navy into whose guns so much of the iron was made, explain the origins of the industry.

There are two methods of extracting iron from its ore – bloomeries and blast furnaces. In Roman times and the early Tudor period, bloomeries were the only available method. These were made by building a mound of alternating layers of ore and charcoal over a shallow pit, covering it with clay and setting it alight. The iron settles as a not quite liquid mass at the bottom of the bloomery and can be extracted when the bloomery is cool. Because this is a batch process requiring the rebuilding of the bloomery for each batch, productivity is quite low.

In the fifteenth century the use of blast furnaces, usually referred to simply as furnaces, gradually superseded bloomeries entirely. With a furnace the raw materials, ore and charcoal, are fed in continuously at the top while iron

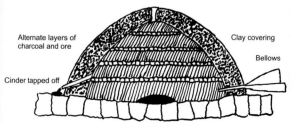

Alternate layers of charcoal and ore

Clay covering

Bellows

Cinder tapped off

Semi-molten iron collected at bottom

Conjectural diagram of a bloomery
(from "Wealden Iron" by Ernest Straker)

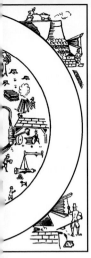

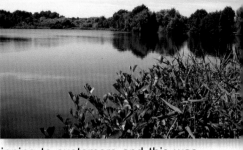

Furnace pond near Horsmonden

and slag are extracted at the bottom. Although this method requires more fuel for a given amount of end product, the much higher productivity ensured its universal adoption.

The "sows" of iron produced by the furnace required further processing before shipping to customers and this was done in a forge where the sows were heated to reduce carbon content and hammered to remove residual slag. A lot of power was required to drive the hammers and as this was usually derived from water wheels most forges were near rivers. To secure supplies of water, large ponds were constructed and many "hammer ponds" can still be found enhancing the Wealden landscape.

The furnaces too required power to drive the bellows that pumped in air and perusal of the map will reveal that many "furnace ponds" also remain. Furnaces and forges were rarely located together, possibly to avoid competition for limited supplies of water power, so transportation between the two was necessary.

Much wood was required for the charcoal so woodland had to be managed sustainably, often by coppicing with a cycle of around 16 years between harvests. Much coppice remains in the Weald, used now for fence posts and fuel rather than for charcoal, although often management has been neglected in recent years.

By far the largest part of the cost of producing iron was the cost of the charcoal. When coke, not then available in Kent and Sussex, became the preferred source of fuel and carbon for producing iron, Wealden iron became uncompetitive. By 1775 the industry was in steep decline and by 1830 it had gone completely. Many vestiges of its former glory remain to be spotted by those who look, often just by studying the map. They are a large part of what gives the area its special character and one wonders how current attempts to exploit the area's natural resources will be viewed in another 300 years.

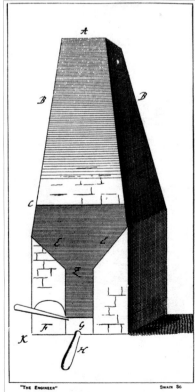

"THE ENGINEER"   SWAIN SC

Gloucester Furnace, Lamberhurst.
From Swedenborg's " De Ferro," 1724.

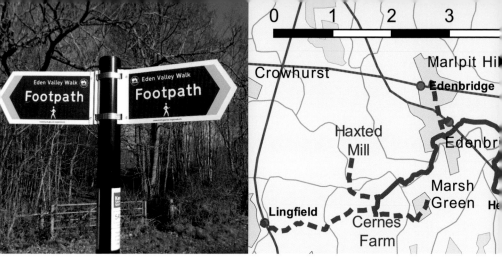

Eden Valley Walk

Introduction

The Eden Valley is very rural and in the past has seen prosperity from iron production in Tudor times, from agricultural production for the London market and from the leather industry. Human occupation has a long history. There was an Iron Age camp at Dry Hill (a couple of miles south of Cernes Farm) and Edenbridge High Street was originally part of the Roman road from London to Lewes, built partly to transport the products of the even earlier Roman iron industry.

The Eden Valley Walk is not everywhere maintained and waymarked to the highest standard, especially west of Hever. Public transport can be a bit haphazard too, especially at weekends. We have tried to provide sufficient information and description of options to enable you to take full advantage of a very attractive route despite these shortcomings.

Itinerary Options

The walk starts at Cernes Farm, a couple of miles west of Edenbridge, and finishes at Tonbridge Castle; east of Penshurst it is following the Medway rather than the Eden Valley.

Some may choose to complete the 15-mile walk in a day but the logistics of getting to the starting point and returning from Tonbridge would make the day a long one.

The starting point at Cernes Farm is quite remote with no access by public transport or private car. When the route of the EVP was originally published back in the late 1980s, two link routes to Cernes Farm were offered.

One of these was from Haxted Water Mill which in those days was a water mill museum and restaurant with a car park that the owners kindly made available to those walking the EVP. The museum, restaurant and car park are long gone and there is no satisfactory parking near the mill. There are no buses either

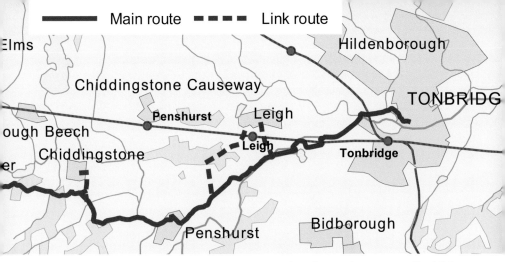

Main route ▬▬▬▬ Link route

Elms
Hildenborough
Chiddingstone Causeway
TONBRIDG
Penshurst   Leigh
ough Beech
Leigh
Chiddingstone   Tonbridge
er
Bidborough
Penshurst

and the road from Edenbridge is too busy and fast for a pleasant walk. This link route is probably useful only if arriving in Edenbridge by train and taking a taxi to the mill.

The second link route offered is a walk from Lingfield station. This is a much better option as the walk is a very pleasant 2.4 miles and is described later. You can return from Edenbridge to Lingfield by bus (25 minutes journey time but buses only every couple of hours or more and none at weekends) or train (there is a train every hour or so but you have to change at Hurst Green (the one in Surrey, not East Sussex) so the journey takes just over an hour). A return journey from Hever Station by train is just a few minutes longer.

Perhaps a more useful and more attractive link route than that from Haxted Water Mill is one from Marsh Green and a description is provided here. There is plenty of parking near the old schoolhouse and there is a bus service, albeit not very frequent and not at weekends.

If you are travelling entirely by public transport then a possible itinerary is as follows:

> Day 1: Lingfield Station – Cernes Farm – Edenbridge – Hever Station (7.3 miles)
>
> Day 2: Hever Station – Penshurst: take bus to either Penshurst Station (which is at Chiddingstone Causeway) or Edenbridge (no bus on Sundays)
>
> Day 3: Leigh – Penshurst – Tonbridge then bus or train back

If using a car, the following is suggested:

> Day 1: Park in Edenbridge, get bus to Marsh Green, walk to Cernes Farm then back to Edenbridge and on to Hever Station (6.5 miles), take train back to Edenbridge
> OR

park in Marsh Green, walk to Cernes Farm then Edenbridge and Hever Station and walk back to Marsh Green (about 9 miles in total, depending on route back from Hever – a possible route is shown in orange dots although it does mean walking the bit between Lydens Farm and Hever Station twice in order to "bag" the entire route)

Day 2: Park at Chiddingstone, walk to Hever Station along orange dotted route and back along the Eden Valley Walk (about 7 miles in total)

Day 3: Park at Penshurst, walk to Chiddingstone along orange dotted route and back along the Eden Valley Walk

Day 4: Park near the green at Leigh, walk to Penshurst (possible route shown in orange) and on to Tonbridge then bus or train back to Leigh

Cycling

There is no special provision for cyclists on the route west of Penshurst. From Penshurst to Tonbridge there is an excellent cycle track, the Tudor Trail. It is also possible with a mountain or hybrid bike to cycle along the bridleway that runs from the minor road west of Wat Stock past Gilridge to Penshurst – but do remember always to give way to walkers. However loud your bell, never assume you've been heard – some walkers are deaf.

Link Route from Lingfield Station to Cernes Farm

The trickiest bit of the journey occurs as soon as you get off the train. If the footpaths on the definitive map were all open you would just leave the station on the west side of the railway, turn left down a path between fences parallel to the railway and at the end turn left across the railway by a path over a pedestrian level crossing. At the time of writing, however, the level crossing has been closed for safety reasons since 2011 after two girls using the crossing were only just missed by a train. The current diversion involves instead crossing the line by the footbridge at the station, walking along the downside (east) platform and taking a short path to the east side of the crossing. If, as is likely, you are on the downside platform when you get off the train, this is actually quite convenient.

There have been various attempts to find a permanent solution. Network Rail tried initially to make the current temporary diversion permanent but this was rejected by Surrey County Council. Network Rail then proposed a new footbridge about halfway along the platform but this was also rejected (in December 2017) because it had only steps (no ramps or lift) and was therefore unsuitable for people with disabilities and parents with children in prams and buggies. Eventually something will change but probably not soon.

Whatever the means by which you get to the east side of where the pedestrian level crossing used to be, now walk eastwards away from the railway and bear slightly right along the right hand edge of one field to a footbridge and across another to a second footbridge. Bear slightly right along a track between two fields to a junction of four paths. There should be a path going across the middle of a field on your left; the path you want is at right angles to this, uphill along the right hand edge of the field.

In the next field the path follows the curving right hand edge and at the corner enters woodland through a slightly off-putting metal gate. Bear slightly left then right through the wood, passing various structures some of which are presumably an outdoor gym for NCYPE, then leave the wood through more metal gates. Bear slightly left over a stile then across a couple of fields to a lane.

Bear left across the lane to a path that soon follows the left hand edge of a playing field. Near the end take a stile and a concrete footbridge over a ditch into a field and follow the right hand edge. Follow the right hand edges of two fields and at the corner turn left along two more right hand field edges to a footbridge in the corner. Over the bridge, follow yet two more right hand field edges. Cross the next field diagonally to the top corner, follow track to drive of Starborough House, turn right to concrete farm track and right along track to lane.

Take track opposite and follow until it bears right at Starborough Manor. Go through gate straight ahead and turn sharp left along track towards Cernes Farm. In small field just before the farm are two finger posts bearing Vanguard Way markers. The second of these marks the start of the Eden Valley Way, although there is currently nothing on it to say so.

NCYPE

The link route passes through the grounds of The National Centre for Young People with Epilepsy, now operating as Young Epilepsy.

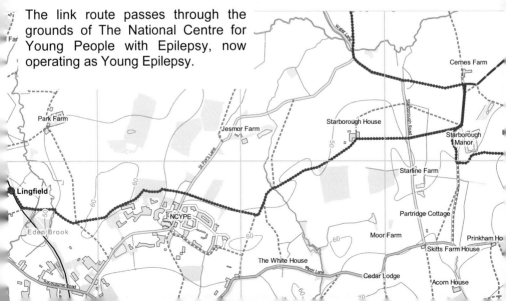

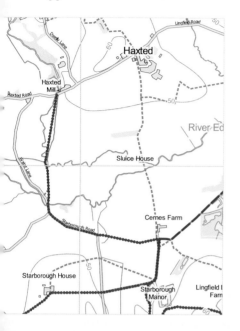

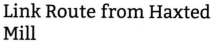

Link Route from Haxted Mill

Take path over stile immediately before the brickwork of the bridge parapet. Head south with hedge on left and river on right until you reach a footbridge over the Eden. On the far side bear just a little left and make for the road bridge over Eden Brook. Just before the bridge climb some wooden steps to a stile onto lane, turn left over the bridge and left again at junction of lanes.

Follow lane for 400m to sharp right hand bend and go over the stile on the corner. Take path gradually moving away from hedge on right and go over stile at far side about 50m to the left of the right hand corner. Cross next field and go through kissing gate to reach the finger post that marks the start of the Eden Valley Walk.

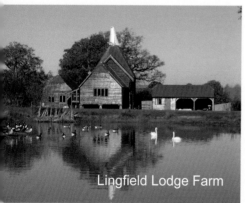

Lingfield Lodge Farm

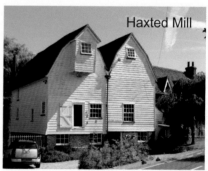

Haxted Mill

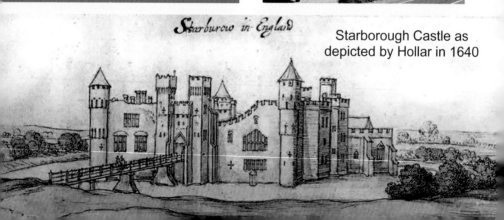

Starborough Castle as depicted by Hollar in 1640

Points of Interest

Haxted Mill

There has been a watermill on the site at least since 1361. The present mill was built in 1580 with substantial additions in 1794. A Mr Woodrow bought the mill in 1949 and spent 20 years restoring it to full working order. For a time there was a museum at the mill and from 1985 until 2014 it housed a popular restaurant but both are now closed.

The water wheel at the front of the building is perhaps more decorative than functional.

Starborough Castle

The original medieval castle built in the 1340s was as large as Bodiam Castle in Sussex. It was demolished in 1648, soon after the execution of Charles I, on the orders of Oliver Cromwell who feared occupation by Royalists. Sir James Burrows, twice President of the Royal Society, used materials from the demolished castle in 1754 to build a modest gothic "pavilion" with battlements on the island in the moat. This two-bedroomed property has fallen into disrepair and been restored more than once and in 2017 was on sale for £1.75m along with additional accommodation in a nearby cottage and a narrow boat moored in the moat. The much larger house visible from the public footpath to the south is a mansion built beside the moat in 1870.

Link Route from Marsh Green to Cernes Farm

Park on the side road near the old school. Go to the main road, cross and turn right. Follow the footway until it ends. Turn left up Greybury Lane. Opposite a row of houses on the left, take path over stile on right downhill through woods to road. Take path opposite.

Follow path through wood to join track at T-junction. Turn right but shortly take path on left before large pond at Lingfield Lodge Farm. Follow path between fences then across large open field. Cross small footbridge and follow path around edge of Starborough Castle with glimpses of old moat and fine Victorian house.

On reaching asphalt drive, take path opposite, turning right along field edge parallel to drive. At corner emerge onto concrete track and turn right to gate ahead. Turn sharp left along track towards Cernes Farm. In small field just before the farm are two finger posts bearing Vanguard Way markers. The second of these marks the start of the Eden Valley Walk, although there is nothing on it to say so.

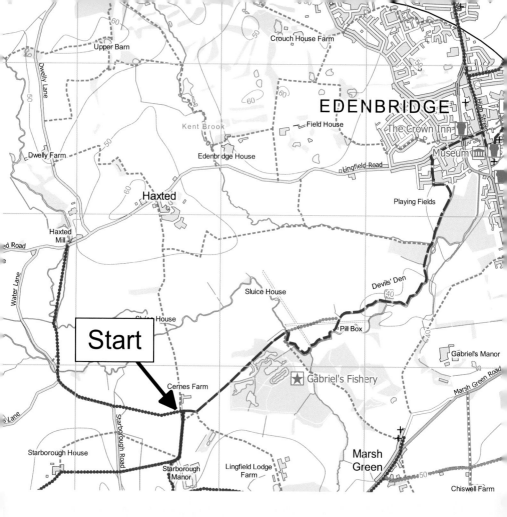

Cernes Farm to Hever Station (4.9 miles)

The walk starts in a small grassy area adjacent to the farm access track immediately south of Cernes Farm. There are two wooden finger posts and the starting point for the walk is the post closest to the farm although it makes no reference to the walk.

With Cernes Farm on your left, head away from the track across rough grassy area to stile in left hand corner then bear left across pasture to stile beside a field gate. Over stile, follow broad track with ponds of Gabriel's Fishery on right, some rather overgrown, to rough grassy area used as parking for the fishery. Go straight ahead to footbridge and cross the Eden.

There is a grass airstrip here. The official route of the EVW goes immediately right along the riverbank. However in early summer the riverside path may be very lost in the lush grass that attracts so many butterflies and dragonflies and there

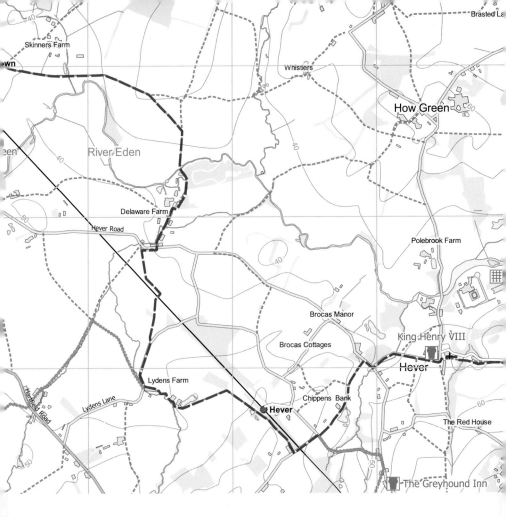

is a well-used path across the airstrip shown in orange on the map. An outline of the mown area of the airstrip is shown but this may be different at the time of your visit. The routes join up at the rusty iron framework.

For the official route, turn sharp right along riverside path and follow round a left hand bend with grass airstrip on left. After a couple of hundred metres bear left, passing pill box on your right, to gap in hedge marked by an iron framework that is apparently part of a bridge (and may rust away before too many years have passed) and continue with hedge on your right.

Soon pass Devil's Den on left and follow riverside path to enter large recreation ground. Follow right hand edge of ground – don't be tempted by paths on right leading into recently restored water meadows. At the corner, where there is a curious iron structure, the official route turns left to car park entrance then right and along Coomb Fields to Haxted Road, right to the crossroads and ahead to the High Street at the other side.

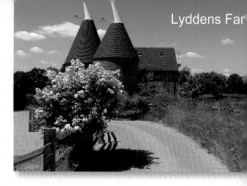
Lyddens Far

Alternatively and more pleasantly, at the iron structure (made to help the tug-of-war team practice) turn right and at an information board for the Great Stone Bridge Trust climb the bank on the left. Turn right, cross relief road and head for the High Street.

There are plenty of opportunities for refreshment here but to continue the walk find Church Street and head for the church. Go through lych gate into church yard. Follow broad path to left of church, bearing right at corner along edge of cemetery to emerge in Churchfield. Bear right to end, turn right into Forge Croft and almost immediately left along broad uphill track over railway. At end cross small parking area, go through small gate and bear right into field. Follow left hand edge of field and at corner turn right along field edge. Follow left hand edge of this and next field then cross bridge over ditch. Go straight ahead up next field to gate then bear slightly right to pass to right of clump of trees and stile at top.

Over stile, bear right diagonally downhill across field to join track at corner; turn right along track downhill to bear left through metal kissing gate and cross the Eden. Follow track around Delaware Farm then turn left

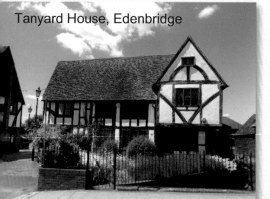
Tanyard House, Edenbridge

along drive to Hever Road. Take path immediately opposite which turns right parallel to road. When hedge bears right, go through gate on left and bear left to far edge of field (not the path that goes straight across and meets the far edge at right angles but one about 45 degrees left of that which may not be apparent on the ground). Turn left along field edge below railway embankment and follow to gate on right leading to tunnel under railway. On the other side of the tunnel, bear diagonally left across field to barrier at far corner. Turn right along lane.

At Lyddens Farm turn left along track with recently restored oast houses on left and converted barn on right. Go through small gap between converted barn on right and garage on left then bear left up path through garden to gate onto track. Turn right along track keeping to right of all farm buildings. At a pair of field gates, turn left over stile between them and along edge of fenced area on left containing trees and pond. Past fenced area, go straight ahead across field making for right hand edge of wood at far side. Here turn right but gradually bear left towards fence alongside railway line. Go through kissing gate on left and either keep right along path parallel to railway to lane or bear left down to footbridge at Hever station.

Points of Interest Between Cernes Farm and Hever Station

Cernes Farm

A listed early 16th century building with 17th century extensions. It is timber-framed with whitewashed brick cladding and hung tiles.

Gabriel's Fishery

The lakes and surrounding woodland are man-made, created in the early years of the 20th century on what was previously arable farmland and meadow. In 2012 the development was presented with an award by Kent Wildlife Trust for its contribution to wildlife diversity, especially wildflowers, birds and butterflies.

East Haxted Farm Airstrip

Apparently used for microlights. There is an air accident report of an incident in July 2016 when a 90 year-old pilot attempting to abort a landing in turbulent conditions found himself and his microlight in an oak tree some five metres above ground from where he had to be rescued by the emergency services.

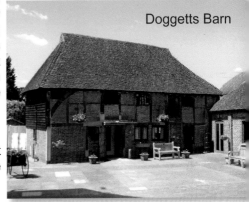

Doggetts Barn

Devil's Den

There are the shallow remains of a moat around the site which may once have contained a farmstead.

Edenbridge

Straddling the old Roman road from London to Lewes, the town was originally called "Eadhelmsbrigge" (Eadhelm's Bridge) and gave its name to the river rather than the other way round. Eadhelm was an abbot from Canterbury who ordered the building of the first proven bridge here in 1125. There are plenty of pubs, a museum and some fine old buildings such as Doggetts Barn, now the home of Edenbridge Town Council.

From the 15th century until 1974, leather production was a major activity in the town. The river provided the needed quantities of water while the bark of the oaks that grow so well on the clay of the Low Weald provided the tannin.

Hever Station

The station was the scene of the Mark Beech riots in 1866 when English navvies attacked lower-paid French workers during the construction of the railway line.

Hever Station to Penshurst (4.9 miles)

Cross the footbridge, take the path up the embankment and turn left along the top to the lane. Turn left to T-junction with two gateways opposite.

Take the path between fences to the right of both gates, passing lake on right and large house on left (Chippen's Bank). On reaching Hever Road turn right then take first left and continue to Henry VIII public house.

Round corner, enter churchyard, take path to right of church, out of churchyard, past some buildings then alongside fence with drive to Hever Castle car park on the other side. At car park, bear sharp right, climb to cross footbridge over driveway and emerge onto broad grassy verge beside driveway. Follow verge round to left. At turning area in front of houses, take path half right between fences (through small wicker gate – easy to miss) and follow to lane.

Take path opposite along field edge then bearing right over bridge across stream (see Points of Interest). Soon bear sharp left over another stream then follow path uphill through woods. Cross wide ride then at skewed T-junction turn left along bridleway. Follow sunken track between fine outcrops of sandstone then emerge

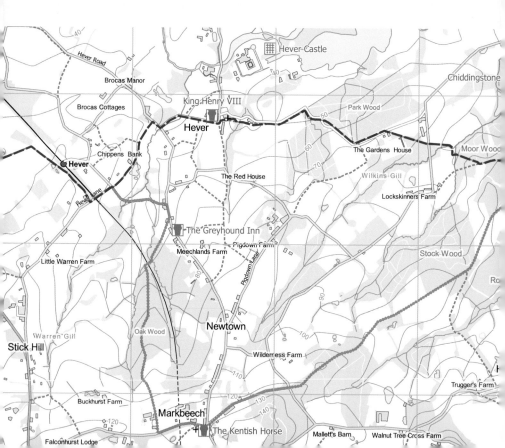

onto lane at Hill Hoath noting Withers (see Points of Interest) on your left.

At first bend take farm track on right then bear left between farm buildings and along path between fences. At the end of a pond on left, take grassy track on right downhill towards woodland[1]. Follow broad track through woodland to lane.

Turn right but soon take path on left through gate and across meadow to farm track. Turn left then left at bend. After a few metres do not take track on right but go forward along track soon becoming rough between hedges. Continue for around one kilometre, possibly passing fruit growing in polytunnels, to meet a concrete farm track. Turn left across bridge over the Eden and uphill to main road at Penshurst.

Turn left and after 100 metres or so take path through metal kissing gate on right. Double back at 45 degrees to road heading directly for church tower. At corner of parkland go through gate into churchyard. Keep to right of church and bear right under overhanging buildings into small courtyard known as Leicester Square. Descend steps and turn left to arch over entrance to Penshurst Place (or turn right to visit Leicester Arms or tearooms).

_____

[1] Or go straight on then left at far side of copse for detour to Chiddingstone

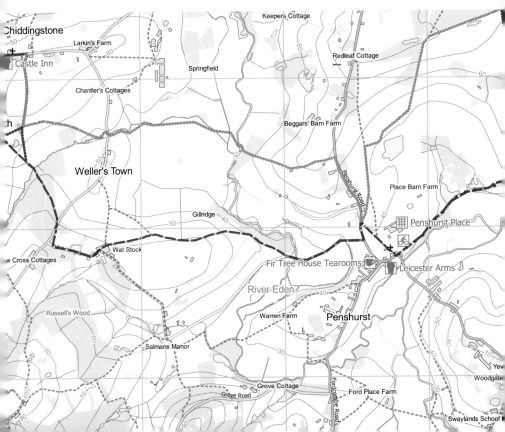

Points of Interest Between Hever Station and Penshurst

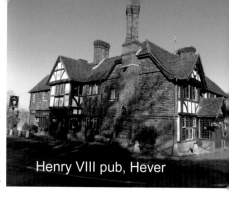

Henry VIII pub, Hever

Chippens Bank

In the early twentieth century the house and model farm were the home of Ethel Everest, daughter of the surveyor after whom the Himalayan mountain is named. Here she would host visits by students from London's Morley College and from London's slum dwellers, the latter organised by Emma Cons and her niece Lilian Baylis who later became a renowned theatrical producer.

Henry VIII Pub

The building proudly sports the date 1597 but apparently that is the date of the first inn on the site, the present building dating from 1647. The parish records supposedly state that the inn was originally called the "Bull 'n' Butcher" and given its present name in 1848; however, when the author Richard Church passed this way in the 1940s he referred to it as the "Boleyn Arms". In the 1980s the pub was owned by a gangster associate of the Crays, George Francis, who in 1985 was shot while behind the bar. He survived only to be killed by a gunman in East London in 2003. Fear not, the pub is respectable and welcoming to walkers now.

Hever Castle

Built in 1462 by Thomas Bullen (Boleyn) whose daughters Anne and Mary became Henry VIII's wife and mistress respectively. The castle was the

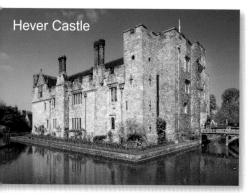

Hever Castle

principal home of Anne of Cleves for the seventeen years from the annulment of her marriage to Henry VIII until her death in 1557, after which it fell into decay. It was bought in 1903 by American millionaire William Waldorf Astor who carefully restored it and had the lake created. He also built the Tudor-style village to provide additional luxury accommodation, now used for conferences and other events.

Old Bridge

The bridge over a stream just before reaching Moor Wood is a far more substantial structure of brick and sandstone than a rural path would justify and is thought to have carried an old coach road from Hever to Penshurst which would very likely have followed an already established route. Henry VIII may well have come this way if, as suggested by the Penshurst Place web site, he stayed at Penshurst (which he owned and used as a hunting lodge) while courting Anne Boleyn. Much of the walk from Hever to Penshurst may follow the old coach road.

Sandstone Outcrop

Shortly before reaching Hill Hoath the path passes between fine outcrops of Ardingly sandstone which was laid down in a river delta about 135 million years ago. It is particularly resistant to weathering, other outcrops of the same stone in the south east being very popular with climbers. It is tempting to interpret the corridor-like route as the remains of an ancient trackway worn down by the passage of people and vehicles across the centuries and some writers have done so. However, careful examination of the rock faces reveals chisel marks; perhaps the stone was quarried for building, perhaps it was removed to create part of the old coach road or perhaps both.

Withers at Hill Hoath

Grade II listed fifteenth century timber-framed building, probably a hall house, once housing the village laundry. According to the Historic England listing, the front has a tile-hung first floor while the rear shows exposed framing with plaster infill, so the side facing the path must be the rear. The ground floor of red brick is nineteenth century infill; the pattern of blue headers (the ends of the bricks are exposed) is known as diaper.

Chiddingstone

Claimed by some to be the prettiest village in Kent, Chiddingstone boasts a 14th century church (much restored after a fire in 1624) and an unspoiled row of 16-17th century houses, many half-timbered or tile-hung, much used for films and television dramas.

The nearby Chiding Stone may or more probably may not have given the village its name. The stone may or may not have been used by villagers as a place to chide wrongdoers and nagging wives.

Chiddingstone Castle

Once the manor house and belonging to the Streatfeild family for many centuries, their wealth stemming from the Wealden iron industry, it was rebuilt in 1679 in a pseudo-medieval style. The main street which used to run past the manor was blocked off and diverted round the castle grounds. The castle is open to the public in the summer months from Sunday to Wednesday and there is a tea room that can be visited without paying for admission to the castle.

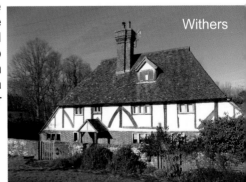
Withers

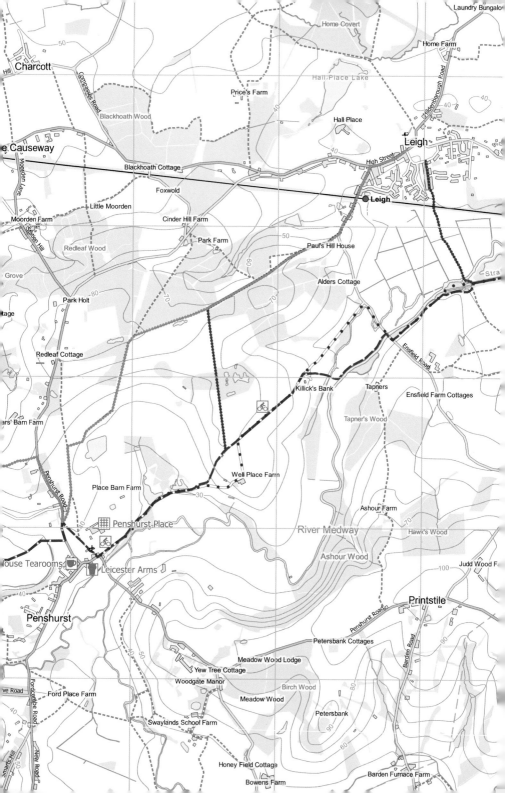

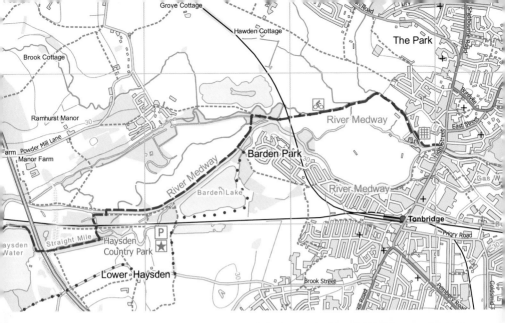

Penshurst to Tonbridge Castle (5.2 miles)

Go through the archway leading to the Penshurst Place car park. Continue along the asphalt drive past the car park and some fish ponds on the left and take a path on the left just before the drive starts to climb steeply. Initially follow the hedge then bear left to a stile at the top of the hill. Through the stile, soon join a concrete track and keep straight ahead descending gradually to reach a group of buildings on the right at Killick's Bank. At junction of tracks here go over stile on right, across pasture and downhill across small footbridge over a stream to bank of the Medway. Bear left along river bank to road.

Turn right across bridge over Medway then take cycle track on left. Follow track between hedge and fence until it starts to bear left into woodland; go through stile on right and follow left hand edge of field to end. Go over stile and then through stile on left into woodland. Turn right along straight track (water-filled cutting on left is westerly part of the "Straight Mile"). At end where there is a wildlife reserve with restricted access straight ahead, turn left over James Christie Bridge.

Follow track with Haysden Water on your right and soon the Medway on your left. When the Medway goes under the arched railway bridge, turn right between the railway on your left and Haysden Water on your right. Just before reaching the A21 viaduct crossing high above, turn right with the viaduct on your left and Haysden Water on your right. Just before reaching a flood defence embankment ahead, turn left along the right hand edge of a water filled ditch. At end of ditch climb embankment and descend the other side without change of direction. Look for path alongside the easterly section of the "Straight Mile" – there should be a waymark, the remains of the canal should be on your

50

left and there should be another ditch on your right used as a bridleway.

Take first bridge, an elegant wooden structure called the Straight Mile Bridge, on left. On reaching railway ahead, go under the railway arch and on the other side straight ahead to a T-junction. Take first bridge on left, the Friendship Bridge, over the Medway and turn right along riverside path. Pass but don't cross Lucifer Bridge, a fine metal lattice, and continue across two more bridges to a T-junction. Turn right and follow footpath, with cycle track close by and sometimes crossing the footpath, under railway bridge and alongside meadows.

On entering car park go straight ahead to entrance of Tonbridge swimming pool then turn sharp left over bridge into park. Turn right and continue to High Street where the walk ends – and the Medway Valley Walk begins.

Points of Interest between Penshurst and Tonbridge

Penshurst Place

Said to be the finest medieval mansion in Kent, Penshurst Place has since 1552 been the home of the Sidney family. It was previously owned by the Stafford family, the Dukes of Buckingham, but the last in the line was beheaded, the house was confiscated by the Crown and given to Sir William Sidney for his loyal service. The most famous of the Sidneys, Sir Philip, was born here in 1554 and became a poet and soldier in the time of Elizabeth I.

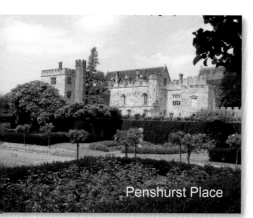
Penshurst Place

The house boasts a Great Hall dating from the 14th century, an Armoury, a Tapestry Room and a Long Gallery. There is a tea room, the Porcupine Pantry, that can be visited without paying for admission to the house. A porcupine has long been a feature of the Sidney coat of arms.

Hall Place (Leigh)

The present house was built from 1871-76 by Samuel Morley, an industrialist, MP and supporter of the temperance movement who had bought the estate in 1870. Many houses in Leigh village were built at around the same time and in the same style – with red and blue brickwork in a pattern known as diapering. The house was damaged by fire in 1940 and reduced in size in 1975-76. Morley provided the endowment necessary to found Morley College in London, whose rambling club celebrated its centenary in 2012.

Killick's Bank

A Grade II listed late medieval hall house but sufficiently altered externally for this not to be obvious – in particular the gable rather than a hipped roof at one end suggests that a wing has been demolished.

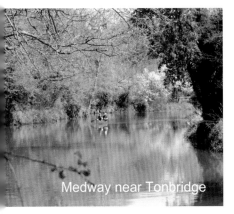

Haysden Water

The Straight Mile

The Medway had been made navigable up to Tonbridge in the 1740s. In 1829 a group led by James Christie set up the Penshurst Canal Company to extend the navigation to Penshurst and beyond. However, legal disputes with the Medway Navigation Company which controlled the section from Medway to Tonbridge and even fighting between the staff of the two companies bankrupted Christie's venture leaving the Straight Mile dug but not filled with water. Christie fled to America leaving huge debts and the Straight Mile is now cut in two by Haysden Water.

Medway near Tonbridge

Haysden Water and Leigh Flood Barrier

Haysden Water is the result of gravel extraction in the 1970s. The 1.3 km long, five metre high earth embankment was built in 1982 to create the Leigh Flood Storage Area which can be used to control the flow of the Medway through Tonbridge and reduce flooding risk at times of high rainfall. Steel gates across the Medway where it flows through the embankment can be closed so that water collects upstream of the barrier, flooding up to 686 acres of pasture west of Haysden Water. The storage capacity is around five million cubic metres of water; on 24 December 2013 water levels were within 10 millimetres of the maximum and water had to be released with some homes flooded as a result.

Tonbridge Castle

Founded in the eleventh century and much of it demolished in the Civil War, the castle's chief surviving feature is the gatehouse – considered one of the finest in the country and now housing council offices including the visitor information centre.

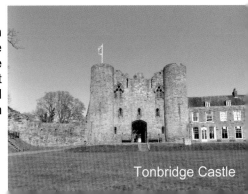

Tonbridge Castle

Medway Valley Walk

Introduction

The Medway is the largest river in Kent, arising in the sandstones of the High Weald and flowing some 70 miles via Tonbridge and Maidstone to Rochester, where it widens and passes Chatham and Gillingham before reaching the Thames. Its main tributaries are the Eden, the Teise and the Beult, the last two joining the Medway near Yalding. The Medway Valley Walk follows only the part of the river downstream from Tonbridge to what was until the opening of the Medway Tunnel the lowest crossing point at Rochester; the Eden Valley Walk follows the Penshurst to Tonbridge part of the Medway Valley.

Planning the Walk

The 28 or so miles of the route from Tonbridge to Rochester can conveniently be divided into four comfortable days using public transport either to and from the starting and finishing points or to get back to a car parked at a starting point.

Tonbridge, Yalding and Maidstone are reasonably well served by trains and so they naturally define the first two sections of the walk. North of Maidstone the railway and path are mainly on opposite sides of the river and only Aylesford station is reasonably accessible from the path. Splitting the route at Aylesford results in a very short third section and a long fourth section and a more even result is obtained by splitting at Burham. The village is half a mile or so from the route but has a small car park and is on a bus route from Rochester to Maidstone.

Cycling the Medway Valley

There is no special provision for cyclists until you reach Barming bridge. From here to Allington Lock the towpath followed by the MVW has been turned into a fine cycle track. From Allington Lock to Aylesford bridge the cycle track continues along the right hand bank of the river while the MVW crosses to the left bank. There is no convenient parking at the Barming end of the track but a good free car park straddles the road at Aylesford. This is not a route for those in a hurry and in places cycles must be pushed rather than ridden.

Piecing together information from the Kent County Council and Sustrans web sites, it seems that a new National Cycle Route 177 is being planned that will connect Rochester to Aylesford as part of a longer route from Northfleet to the south coast via Maidstone and Ashford. Some sections between Aylesford and Wouldham are in place but not enough to be a viable itinerary at the moment. National Cycle Route 17 does run from Maidstone to Rochester but does so via Blue Bell Hill and the North Downs rather than the Medway valley.

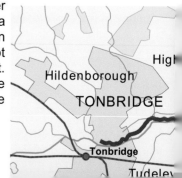

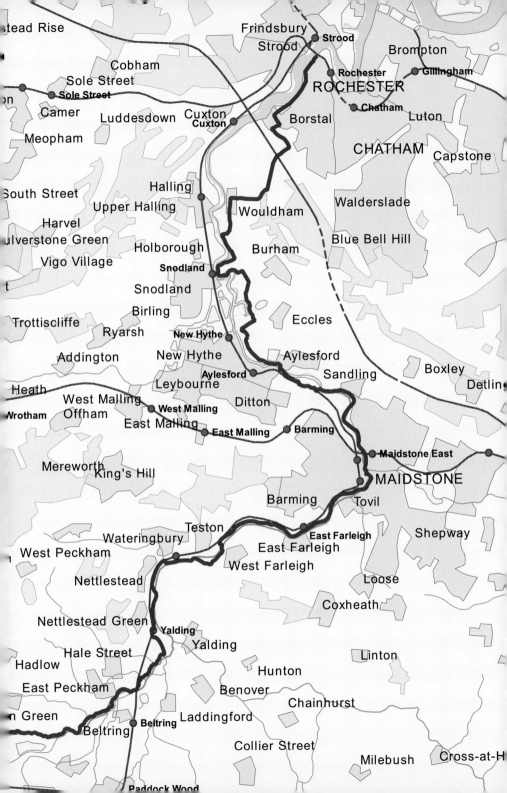

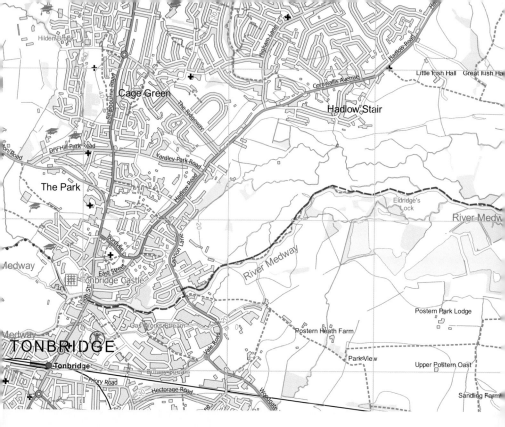

Tonbridge to Yalding Station (8.3 miles)

Start by heading east along Medway Wharf Road. If coming from the railway station, this is the last right turn before the bridge over the Medway. If coming from the castle, it is the first left turn after crossing the river. After the last building on the left, bear left along the river edge and follow the riverside path to the bridge at Vale Road.

Cross the river and take the riverside path on the right. Initially there are some industrial buildings on your left but soon you are out of town with meadows or cropped fields on both sides of the river. Pass under a bridge carrying a rough track to a gravel pit and continue to Eldridge's Lock. Continue to Hartlake Bridge.

Go under the bridge – you should soon be able to see Hadlow Tower to your left and behind it the Greensand ridge – and continue to East Lock. Cross a footbridge to an island, a second footbridge over a weir and a third over the lock itself. Follow the riverside path, the river now on your left, to Ford Green Bridge (a footbridge). Don't cross but continue along the right bank of the river passing Oak Weir Lock and Sluice Weir Lock then an industrial estate to reach Branbridges Road.

Cross the road and take path (see note on map) opposite back to

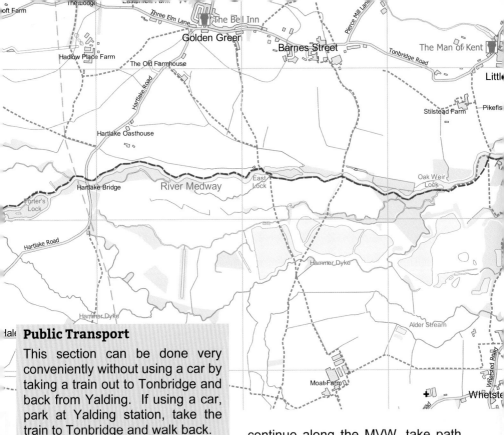

Public Transport

This section can be done very conveniently without using a car by taking a train out to Tonbridge and back from Yalding. If using a car, park at Yalding station, take the train to Tonbridge and walk back.

There is an hourly direct service on weekdays and Saturdays taking only 15 to 20 minutes. On Sundays it is necessary to change at Paddock Wood and the journey takes much longer.

continue along the MVW, take path on right but for the railway station follow the road round to the left and uphill to the station on the right.

riverbank. Pass under a larger bridge carrying the A228. A railway bridge soon follows then a footbridge that you do not cross. Continue along the right bank of the river until you pass a small marina on the right followed by Tea Pot Island and the path bears left across a weir to Hampstead Lane.

Turn left past The Boathouse Inn and alongside the canal. When the road bears left, follow it over the canal. To

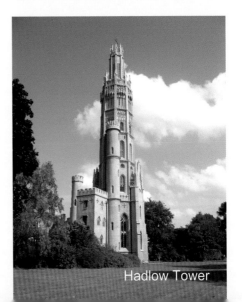

Hadlow Tower

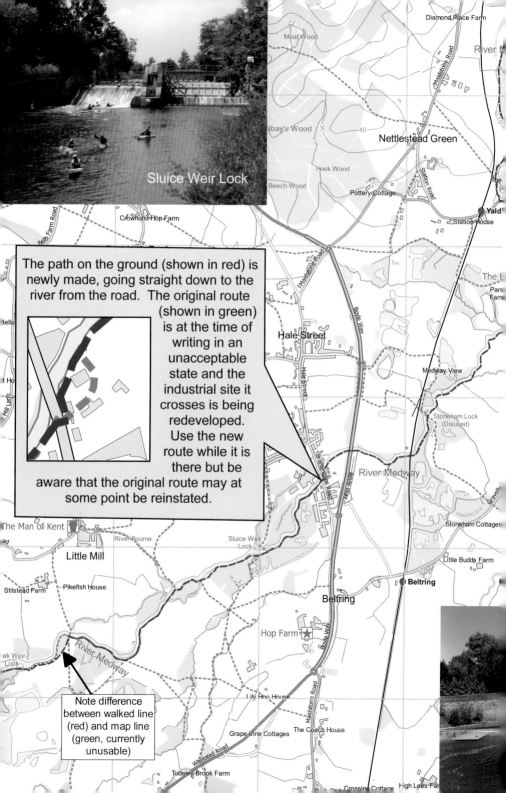

Sluice Weir Lock

The path on the ground (shown in red) is newly made, going straight down to the river from the road. The original route (shown in green) is at the time of writing in an unacceptable state and the industrial site it crosses is being redeveloped. Use the new route while it is there but be aware that the original route may at some point be reinstated.

Note difference between walked line (red) and map line (green, currently unusable)

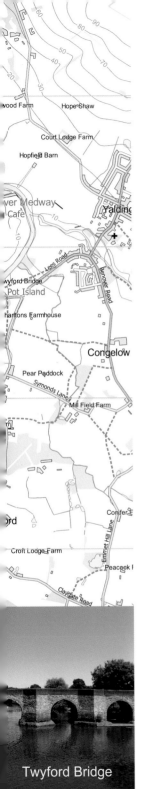

Twyford Bridge

Places of Interest between Tonbridge and Yalding

Tonbridge

Originally spelt "Tunbridge" and still so pronounced, town life centred round the castle until it was largely demolished by the Parliamentarians during the Civil War. Development was stimulated when the Medway became navigable up to the town in 1741 and further when the railway arrived in 1842.

The surviving gateway of the castle is impressive and can be visited; the visitor information centre is adjacent.

Tonbridge has connections to various members of Jane Austen's family, including her father who was a master at Tonbridge School.

Hadlow Tower

This folly was originally part of a neo-Gothic castle completed in 1838 by Walter Barton May. Some say its purpose was to remind May's estranged wife of him wherever she went, some say it was to enable him to spy on her and some say it was intended to give sight of the sea but the challenge of raising it high enough proved too great. The rest of the castle was demolished in 1951 leaving the 150 ft high tower in splendid isolation. It fell into decay but early this century it was superbly restored at huge expense, partly funded by Historic England and the Heritage Lottery Fund. For a while the tower was let as very up-market holiday accommodation and, as a condition of the funding arrangements, opened occasionally to the public. Following the financial failure of the Vivat Trust which undertook the work, the tower is apparently now in private hands and at the time of writing it is not clear that the public opening obligation is being fulfilled.

Hartlake Bridge Disaster

In October 1853 thirty hop-pickers were drowned when a wagon returning them to their camp across the bridge crashed through the wooden side into the swollen river. The coroner found that the cause of the accident was failure by the Medway Navigation Company to maintain the bridge and roadway adequately but the company refused to contribute to the cost of burying the victims in Hadlow churchyard where a monument has been erected.

Hop Farm (Beltring)

Not far away on your right as you approach East Peckham are the oast houses of the former Whitbread Hop Farm although they never quite come into view. Most of the present buildings date from early Victorian times and became known as the 25 cowls of Kent. Whitbread, now better known as owners of Premier Inns and Costa Coffee, were originally brewers and having acquired the farm in 1920 developed it into one of Kent's largest hop farms with over 100 acres devoted to the crop. In 1982 they opened a museum and visitor centre which they sold in the mid-1990s. The venture has since struggled financially under a string of owners but is still operating as both a wedding and conference venue and as a visitor centre offering a variety of attractions including a petting farm, retail outlets and eating places.

Tea Pot Island

A handy place for a cup of tea or an all-day breakfast although opening times should be checked in advance, especially in winter. There is a shop selling an astonishing variety of tea pot designs and an exhibition of tea pots (at extra charge); it is sometimes possible to have a go at making your own.

Yalding

The village of Yalding is half a mile or so from the route of the walk but is worth visiting by detour or separately if time permits. There are some fine old buildings and an exceptionally long medieval bridge over the Beult from which you can look down in early summer onto water meadows carpeted with an excellent display of wild flowers. The parish was once the largest hop-growing parish in Kent.

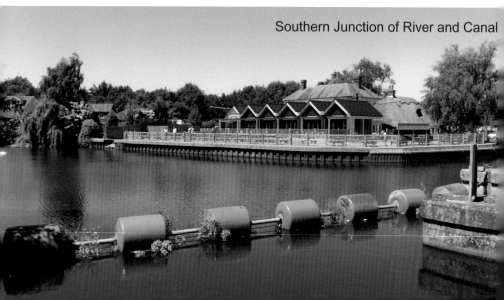

Southern Junction of River and Canal

Hop Growing in Kent

Hop cultivation was introduced into England by Walloon refugees in the sixteenth century and in the latter half of the seventeenth century production expanded rapidly.

Hops belong to the cannabis family of plants and grow prodigiously – up to 20 cm a day. They are cut back each autumn and growth starts afresh in April. A complex system of wires and string is built for the bines to climb up. In the days of hand-picking a height of 4 metres was typical but with machine picking, now universally employed, up to 8 metres is possible.

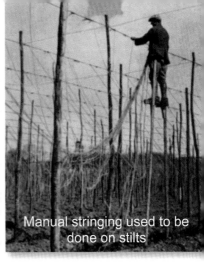

Manual stringing used to be done on stilts

Most hop plants in a garden are female and produce bracts carrying hairs that secrete the yellow resinous lupulin that gives beer its characteristic bitter taste.

Hand picking of hops is very labour-intensive and until the 1960s tens of thousands of Londoners were brought by train into the Kent countryside each September for a hop-picking "holiday". They were housed in primitive conditions in huts, some of which still survive and can be seen as one walks through Kent. Since the early 1960s all hops have been picked mechanically.

The hops then have to be dried and the kilns with their characteristic cowls are a common site although now rarely used for their original purpose. At one time round oast houses were thought to be more efficient but this proved a myth and square kilns became more popular if less picturesque. Despite attempts to ban the practice, brimstone (sulphur) was traditionally burned in the kiln to improve the colour and flavour of the hops.

The Kent hop industry declined calamitously between 1960 and 2000, partly due to the growing popularity of lager and partly due to the plentiful supply of imported hops. In recent years there has been something of a revival thanks to microbreweries, the popularity of "real ale" and a renewed appreciation of the special flavour of English hops.

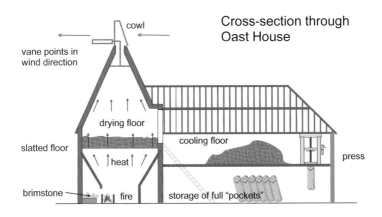

Cross-section through Oast House

cowl

vane points in wind direction

drying floor

slatted floor

heat

brimstone — fire

cooling floor

storage of full "pockets"

press

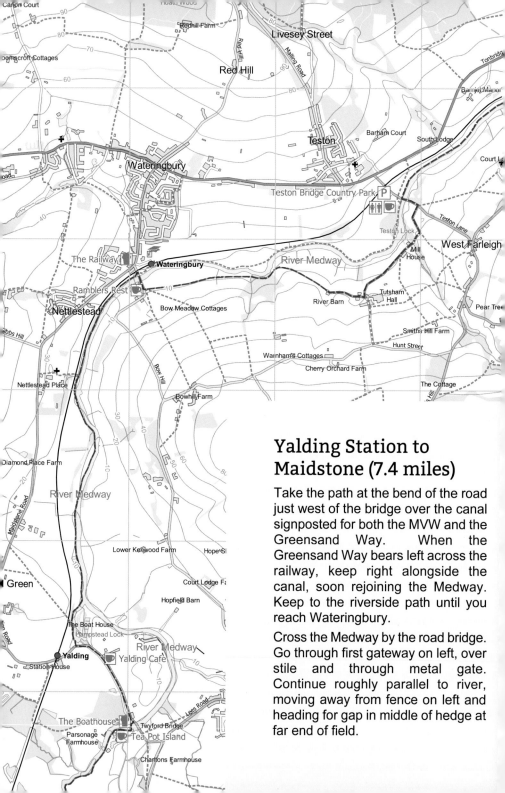

Yalding Station to Maidstone (7.4 miles)

Take the path at the bend of the road just west of the bridge over the canal signposted for both the MVW and the Greensand Way. When the Greensand Way bears left across the railway, keep right alongside the canal, soon rejoining the Medway. Keep to the riverside path until you reach Wateringbury.

Cross the Medway by the road bridge. Go through first gateway on left, over stile and through metal gate. Continue roughly parallel to river, moving away from fence on left and heading for gap in middle of hedge at far end of field.

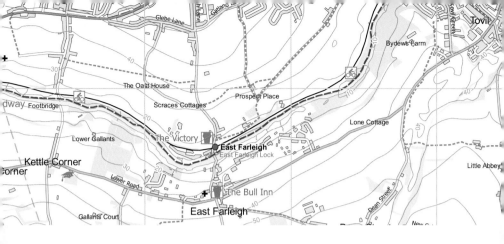

Through gap, gradually approach fence on left and enter a short section of woodland. On the other side bear right uphill and aim for barn at corner of field. Bear slightly left along asphalt track between farm buildings and, at junction in front of Tutsham Hall, go left through kissing gate alongside a cattle grid. Follow track as it bears gently right then past Mill House and cottages with Teston Lock below. Continue along track to Teston Lane, turn left and cross Teston Bridge. On your left is Teston Bridge Country Park with toilets and refreshments but to continue the walk turn right along the river bank.

Follow the riverside path past Barming Bridge (footbridge) and East Farleigh bridge beyond which is a lock. Pass a girder footbridge at Lower Fant and the elegant Lock Meadow Footbridge leading to All Saints' Church but stay on the left bank of the river to the first road bridge carrying Broadway across the river. For Maidstone West station, turn left along Broadway then second left into Station Approach but to continue the MVW take the bridge across the river.

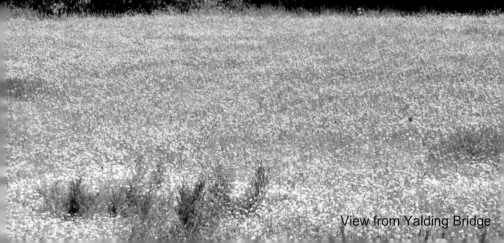

View from Yalding Bridge

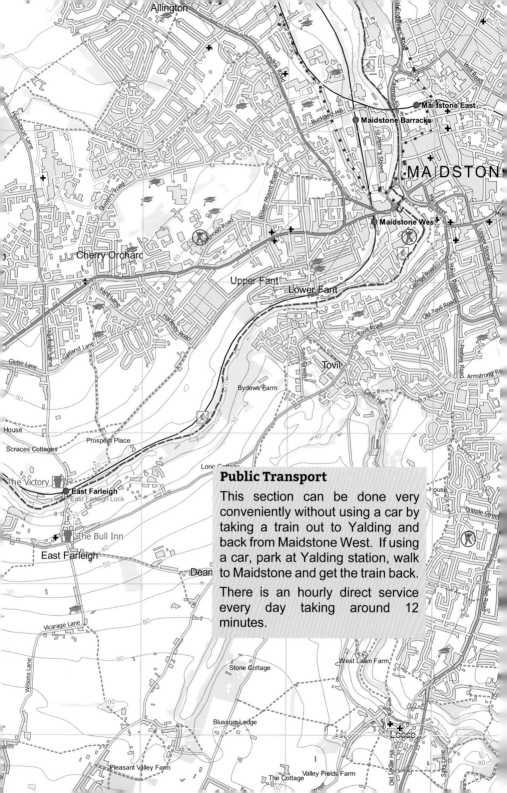

Public Transport

This section can be done very conveniently without using a car by taking a train out to Yalding and back from Maidstone West. If using a car, park at Yalding station, walk to Maidstone and get the train back.

There is an hourly direct service every day taking around 12 minutes.

Points of Interest between Yalding and Maidstone

Rural Rides

In his Rural Ride across Kent from Dover to Westerham in September 1823 William Cobbett described the route from Maidstone to Mereworth thus:

> "From Maidstone to this place (Merryworth) is about seven miles, and these are the finest seven miles that I have ever seen in England or anywhere else. The Medway is to your left, with its meadows about a mile wide. You cross the Medway, in coming out of Maidstone, and it goes and finds its way down to Rochester, through a break in the chalk-ridge. From Maidstone to Merryworth I should think that there were hop-gardens on one half of the way on both sides of the road. Then looking across the Medway, you see hop-gardens and orchards two miles deep, on the side of a gently rising ground: and this continues with you all the way from Maidstone to Merryworth."

The hop-gardens are thinner on the ground nowadays and the road is more built-up in places but the Medway itself and the walk described here retain a very rural feel until they reach Maidstone town.

Kenward House

You will probably notice this house on the far side of the river as you make your way from Yalding to Wateringbury. John Kenward acquired the estate in 1533 and his descendent John Kenward, the last of that surname to own the estate, died in 1749. From 1942 until 1967 the house was a Dr Barnardo's children's home. Since then it has been developed as a Christian centre for rehabilitation of those with alcohol and drug addictions.

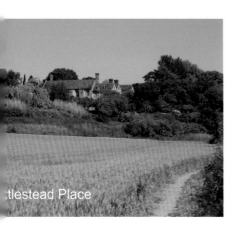

Nettlestead Place

Nettlestead Place

Well-restored 14-15th century house, now a wedding venue. The ten acres of fine gardens are open occasionally under the National Gardens Scheme.

Only the tower of the nearby church of St Mary survives from the original of around 1300, the rest having been rebuilt in the 15th century at the expense of the Pympe family, occupants of Nettlestead Place, to accommodate a collection of stained glass which is widely admired. However the windows were badly damaged by a great storm in 1763 and not all of them were perfectly restored. Simon Jenkins in his book 'England's Thousand Best Churches' describes "the attempt to resolve the jigsaw" as "most casual" and suggests that the right hand window might be a

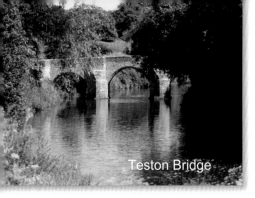
Teston Bridge

"forgery" of 1896 but I can find no other reference to this suspicion.

Wateringbury

Wateringbury seems most famous for a wooden mace known as the "dumb borsholder" which hangs in the church. A borsholder was an elected official and until 1748 it was apparently the practice in the local manor of Chart to elect this mace rather than a human being, although it was given a human deputy to speak on its behalf. It was reported in an Edinburgh review article of 1820 that "this wooden magistrate ... discharged his duties as efficiently as many other country justices".

Teston Country Park

As well as one of the Medway's fine medieval bridges there is a country park with, toilets, refreshment kiosk, picnic tables and parking. There is also a lock.

Barham Court

This gleaming white mansion is prominently visible when looking north from Teston Bridge across the railway. In the 18th century it was described by Kentish historian Edward Hasted (see page 28) as "the greatest ornament of this part of the county". William Wilberforce was a regular guest of Lady Barham and it is thought that a meeting here in 1783 with the local rector, who had been a naval chaplain in the West

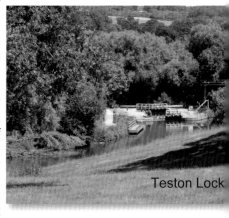
Teston Lock

Indies, kindled his concern to abolish slavery. The property has now been converted into serviced office accommodation.

East Barming

Until 1996 the village's main claim to fame appeared to be the only timber-built vehicular bridge on the Medway which famously collapsed in 1914 when a traction engine was taken across it. In 1996 the bridge was replaced with a less picturesque but stronger steel bridge, also known as Kettle Bridge. This is now also the start of a cycle track beside the

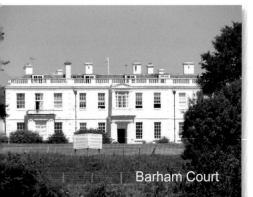
Barham Court

river which was installed around 2017 and continues through Maidstone to Aylesford.

East Farleigh

The village's main claim to fame is its medieval bridge, some say the finest in

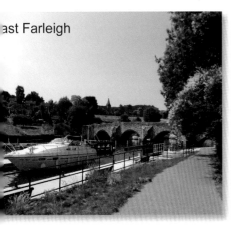

ast Farleigh

southern England. It was over this bridge that General Fairfax led his troops to defeat Royalist forces in Maidstone in 1648. The village has a long history starting in Roman times when ragstone was quarried nearby for use in London buildings. It is mentioned in the Domesday book as "Ferlaga" and in the early 19th century two of William Wilberforce's sons were vicars here. The East Farleigh lock was refurbished at a cost of £3.6 million in 2017 including the installation of a new fish pass providing a climbable slope for freshwater fish to travel upstream.

Maidstone

Maidstone is of course the county town of Kent and although the name is Saxon there has been a settlement here since Roman times. As you enter the town along the riverside you will pass an elegant modern footbridge leading to All Saints Church and the Archbishop's Palace. At the west end of the bridge you may notice a large aluminium sculpture of a stag. This work of art by Edward Bainbridge Copnall was

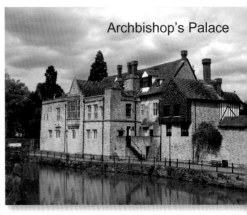

Archbishop's Palace

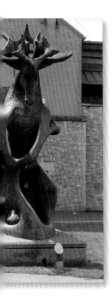

located in Stag Place in London from 1963 until 1997 when the area was redeveloped. The sculpture was then given by Copnall's daughter to Sevenoaks but the District Council was unable to find an appropriate site and controversially sold it to Maidstone Borough Council for £2000.

The Palace once belonged to the Wyatt family but, like Allington Castle, was forfeited to the Crown when Thomas Wyatt the younger rebelled against Mary I.

Maidstone to Burham (6.2 miles plus 0.5 mile link)

Start from the bridge carrying Broadway over the Medway. If coming from Maidstone West station, head downhill to the bridge, cross it and take the steps down to the riverside path. If you are on the upstream side of the bridge, go under the bridge. Follow the path along the right bank of the river going under another road bridge. Climb briefly to the road to go under a railway bridge and return immediately to the river bank. Go under two footbridges and pass Allington marina followed by a brief glimpse of Allington castle on the opposite bank.

At Allington lock, take the footbridge over the weir then cross one of the pairs of lock gates to the left bank. Turn right along path, soon climbing to track. Keep right but then bear left uphill past tracks to boatyard and turn right at top. Take path across railway line with care and turn right through woods until forced to bear left to footbridge over M20. At far side of bridge turn left through woods then into open field. Keep to right hand edge of field with woodland on right then cross gap to more woodland, this time on left. At far side turn right downhill to railway. Turn left alongside railway then at buildings turn right over railway. Turn left along track between railway on left and Medway on right.

On reaching road at Aylesford you may wish to detour briefly onto the ugly modern bridge to admire the much-photographed view of the Medway flowing under the medieval bridge with the church on the hill behind. To continue the walk, however, turn left and take first track on right over the medieval bridge. Turn left along High Street, noting the many fine old buildings.

You can avoid a section without footway by climbing steps on right towards church then left at the top. Continue until road bends sharp right and the entrance to The Friars (Aylesford Priory) is straight ahead. The MVW goes down a concrete track immediately to the right of the Priory entrance but you may wish to detour for refreshment at the Priory tea room.

Heading down the concrete track, note the fine timber-framed and thatched architecture of the old barn housing the Priory tea room over the wall on your left. Keep to the track which soon enters the sewage works and then becomes a pleasant woodland path that bears gently right then sharply left. Follow the path as it approaches then goes around an electricity transmission station graced by some tall pylons. Emerging onto a concrete track, turn right uphill and pass a solar farm on your left. At top bear left and continue until you have passed a large water treatment plant on the left. On reaching a barrier across the track, look for a diagonal path across the fields on the right. If this path is impassable for any reason, you can continue along the concrete track and end up in the same place. When the track and path meet, take an uphill path on the left if you want to go to Burham either to collect your car from the car park or to catch a bus to

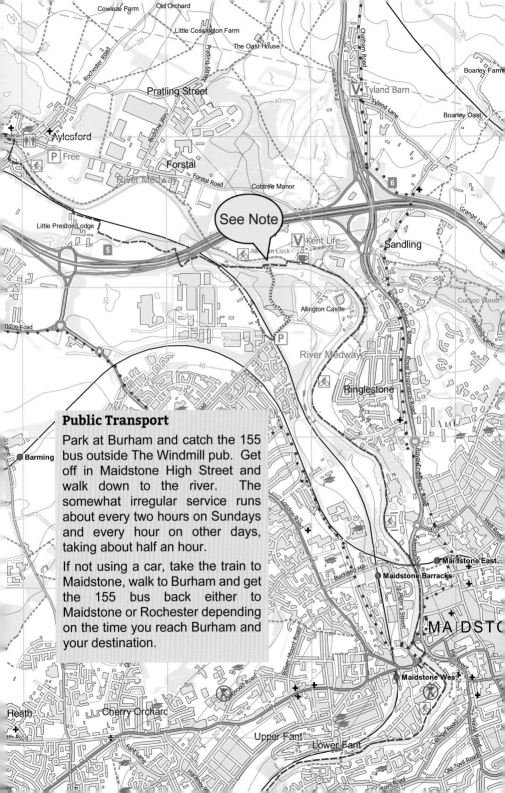

See Note

Public Transport

Park at Burham and catch the 155 bus outside The Windmill pub. Get off in Maidstone High Street and walk down to the river. The somewhat irregular service runs about every two hours on Sundays and every hour on other days, taking about half an hour.

If not using a car, take the train to Maidstone, walk to Burham and get the 155 bus back either to Maidstone or Rochester depending on the time you reach Burham and your destination.

Maidstone or Rochester. To continue along the MVW, bear slightly left along a track towards old Burham church.

Note

The original Kent County Council guide to the MVW and their current on-line map show an alternative route when leaving Allington Lock heading down river. This is shown on the map as a red dotted line and is waymarked with the MVW logo in places whereas the shorter route described above is not. Current KCC staff do not know why this was done and there is no reason to doubt the long-term availability of the direct route. However, the alternative is there if required.

Points of Interest between Maidstone and Burham

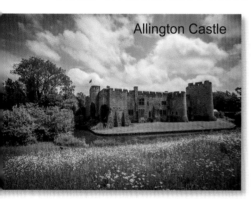
Allington Castle

Allington Castle

Parts date back to early Norman times but most was rebuilt in the late 15th century by Sir Stephen de Penchester and further alterations were undertaken after Sir Thomas Wyatt acquired the castle around 1493. Sir Thomas's son, also Thomas, led a failed revolt against Mary Tudor in 1554; he was executed, Allington was seized, the rest of the family emigrated to America and the castle fell into disrepair.

The mountaineer Lord Conway acquired and restored the castle between 1906 and 1937. From 1951 until 1999 it was occupied by Carmelite nuns under the auspices of the Carmelite Priory that still survives at Aylesford. The castle has been restored yet again by the current owner. It hosts occasional weddings and it is currently possible to visit on a boat trip from Maidstone but it is not otherwise open to the public.

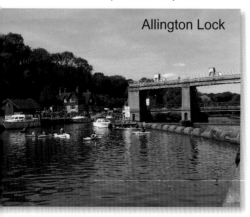
Allington Lock

Allington Lock

The locks upstream of Maidstone are mainly in remote countryside or quiet villages. Allington lock, however, is a bustling venue with a restaurant, a tea-room, many moored boats and often groups of canoeists in brightly coloured life jackets paddling up and down the river above the lock. It is unusual too in having a lock keeper from the Environment Agency which also offers chalet

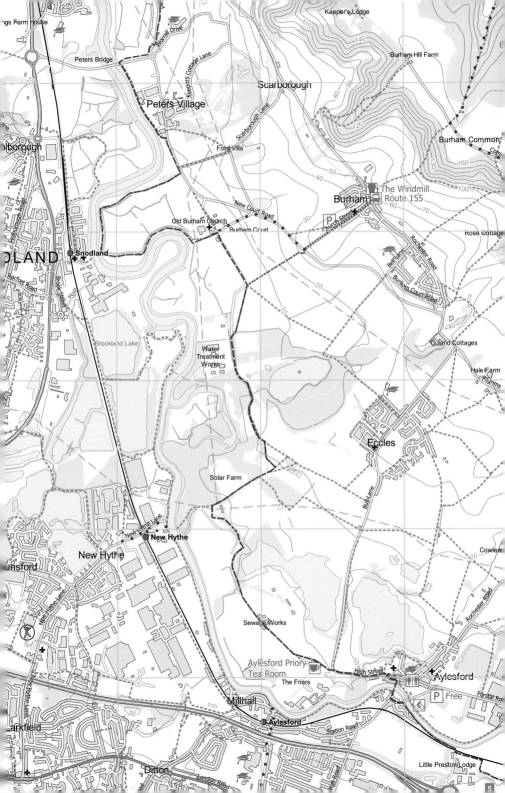

accommodation overlooking the lock for holiday makers.

Kent Life

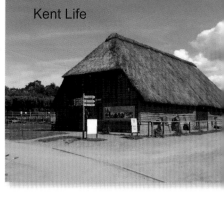
Kent Life

Just two minutes' walk from Allington Lock is Kent Life. Once known as the Kent Museum of Rural Life it was originally Sandling Farm, part of the Allington Castle estate, bequeathed to Maidstone Borough Council in the 1960s. There are reconstructed buildings from other parts of Kent and attractions include an owl academy and a farm animal petting area. The site is now operated on behalf of the Council by a commercial company and the offerings are very much targeted at the younger members of the family.

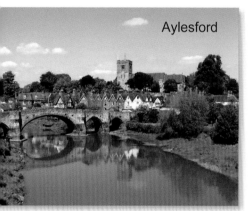
Aylesford

Tyland Barn

Also not far from Allington Lock, although pretty well impossible to visit by a detour on foot thanks to the intervening junction 6 of the M20, is Tyland Barn, headquarters of the Kent Wildlife Trust. There is a free visitor centre with a wildlife garden, cafe and gift shop.

Aylesford

Claimed to be the oldest continuously occupied village, Aylesford owes its antiquity to being the site of the lowest ford across the Medway. In 455 the battle of Aylesford took place here, or perhaps not far away below Bluebell Hill. The invading Jutes under Hengist and Horsa took on the natives under Vortigern, or perhaps his son Vortimer. Possibly the Britons won and possibly they didn't but Horsa died and Hengist went on to certain victory over the Britons at the battle of Crayford in 457.

Built in 1390, the bridge is the oldest on the river but the middle span was enlarged in the 19th century to accommodate the increasing river traffic.

The Friars (Aylesford Priory)

A Carmelite priory was founded here around 1242 when returning crusader Lord Richard Grey provided sites for priories on his estates both here and at

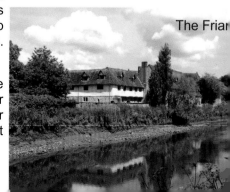
The Friar

Hulne in Northumberland. The Friars were evicted when Henry VIII dissolved the monasteries and the buildings passed into secular hands until reacquired by the Carmelites in 1949. The medieval buildings, some much damaged by a fire in 1930, were restored and a new church built. Many of the buildings are let out for conferences while the grounds are open to the public (no charge apart from parking) with a popular tea room open daily in a thatched 17th century barn.

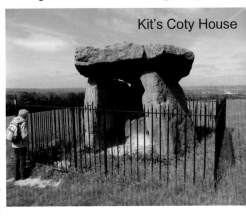

Kit's Coty House

Kit's Coty House

Half way up the North Downs above Aylesford are the remains of a neolithic burial mound or barrow known as Kit's Coty House. The stones now enclosed by iron railings alongside the North Downs Way as it climbs Bluebell Hill are part of a rectangular chamber situated at what used to be the east end of the large, long mound. The path past the site is probably part of the route from Maidstone to Rochester that Charles Dickens described as "one of the most beautiful walks in England". The view from the country park at the top of Bluebell Hill is certainly magnificent but noise from traffic on the A229 does perhaps take the edge off the experience of walking this bit of the North Downs Way.

Not far away but not so easy to access because the entrance is on a busy road is Little Kit's Coty House. This was also a neolithic burial mound but, following demolition in 1690, is now little more than a pile of boulders, hence the alternative name "The Countless Stones".

Blue Bell Hill

A conspicuous feature of the skyline above Aylesford is Blue Bell Hill picnic site, perched on a narrow band of grassland above a huge chalk quarry and offering magnificent views across the Medway valley. There are actually five quarries which expose one of the most complete inland sequences of chalk beds in southern England. The chalk from the quarries was used by Thomas Cubitt as an ingredient in the manufacture of cement, and additional product of his massive brickworks (see Points of Interest for next section). Cement is made by mixing chalk (or limestone) with clay and sand then heating the mixture to nearly 1500° C in a kiln.

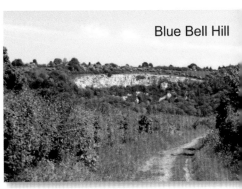

Blue Bell Hill

Burham to Rochester (7.0 miles plus 0.5 mile link)

If starting from The Windmill at Burham, cross the main road, pass the war memorial and head along Church Lane out of the village and down to a T-junction. Take path opposite, down left hand edge of field to join Medway Valley Path at junction with asphalt track. Turn right towards old Burham church which you may choose to visit.

Immediately before the church, turn left along stony track then through gap beside gate along grassy track. At river bank turn right along flood defences and follow round a series of bends with views of Snodland (church and Smurfit Kappa paper recycling plant). You are now walking through the Holborough to Burham Marshes SSSI (see Points of Interest). At your closest point to Snodland church across the river, pass the memorial commemorating the Battle of the Medway where in 43 AD Roman forces defeated the British, although it is by no means certain that this is the correct location. Continue, soon bearing right and then alongside the overgrown remains of the West Kent Portland Cement Works. On reaching

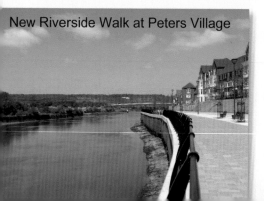

New Riverside Walk at Peters Village

the lane turn left and on reaching the new development of Peters Village bear left along the new riverside walk and cycle track.

Follow the riverside walk past the new development and under the new Peters Bridge over the Medway. Turn right and follow cycle track to lane. Cross at the crossing and turn left past new school and into Wouldham village. Go along High Street through the village and, opposite Rectory Close on the left, take School Lane uphill on right past the old school buildings. Keep going uphill to road at top.

Take uphill track opposite bearing left and right to meet the North Downs Way at a T-junction at the top. Turn left and follow the NDW with open views and fine views across the Medway Valley on your left and narrow strips of woodland on your right. After just over half a mile, bear gently right downhill to bridge over the high speed rail line. Go through Nashenden Farm to T-junction and turn left along asphalt track still following NDW. On meeting road, turn right under the M2 and climb gently into the village of Borstal.

Immediately before Coop store on left, turn left downhill along path between houses. At bottom turn right along path past marina to recreation ground. Keep left through Baty's Marsh nature reserve parallel to river until path meets the road at a corner. Follow the footway along the water's edge and, just before apartment block on left, bear left along riverside walkway. Continue along water's edge until there is a jetty on the left; turn right to road in front of castle then left to the Medway bridge where the walk ends.

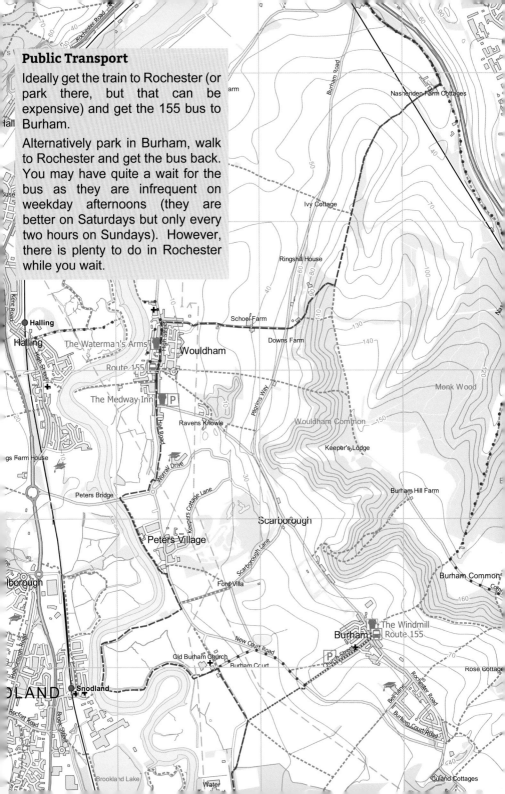

Public Transport

Ideally get the train to Rochester (or park there, but that can be expensive) and get the 155 bus to Burham.

Alternatively park in Burham, walk to Rochester and get the bus back. You may have quite a wait for the bus as they are infrequent on weekday afternoons (they are better on Saturdays but only every two hours on Sundays). However, there is plenty to do in Rochester while you wait.

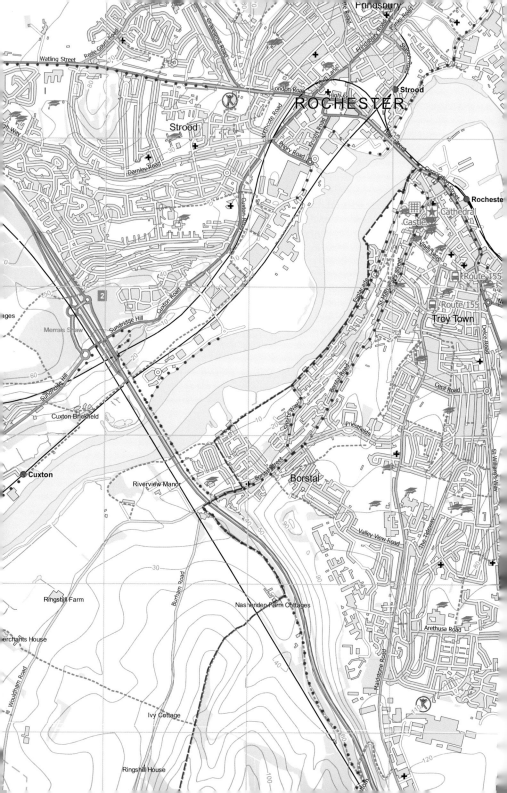

Points of Interest between Burham and Rochester

Burham

The village was originally located around the old church close to the river and adjacent to the MVW. The Domesday Book records 42 households – 15

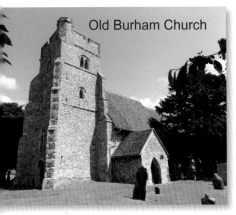

Old Burham Church

villagers, 20 smallholders and 7 slaves. Slavery was common in Anglo-Saxon England but was gradually phased out by the Norman conquerors and by 1120 it was gone.

The village was at a popular crossing point on the Medway for travellers using the Pilgrim's Way, a ferry carrying them to or from nearby Snodland.

The village was transformed in 1852 when Thomas Cubitt established a brickworks here. It was highly mechanised and has been described as the most advanced brickworks in the world, producing up to 30 million bricks a year. Cubitt was an architect and builder responsible for much development in Bloomsbury and for parts of Buckingham Palace and Osborne House. He developed modern, efficient building practices and needed a reliable source of quality bricks. New houses for the workers were built higher up the valley where the Windmill pub and bus stop are now to be found. Few traces of the brickworks now remain.

Holborough to Burham Marshes SSSI

This, the only Site of Special Scientific Interest through which the MVW passes, includes Kent Wildlife Trust's Burham Marsh Nature Reserve. Amongst the reed beds may be lurking kingfisher, cormorant, herons and geese as well as the reed and sedge warbler. Local plants include the marsh mallow.

Wouldham

This is another village listed in the Domesday book that remained largely agricultural until the mid-nineteenth century when a cement factory was built and the population quadrupled to over a thousand. The factory closed in the 1920s as there was no railway on the east bank of the Medway, transportation by barge having become uncompetitive when a new bridge at Rochester

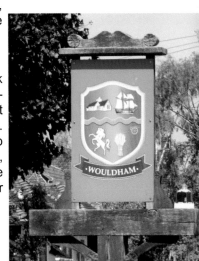

denied sea-going barges access to the river, and all production was transferred to sites on the west bank.

In 2016 a new bridge, the Peters Bridge, was built across the Medway and the sites of the Peters Wouldham Hall Cement Works and Peters Pit are being redeveloped for housing.

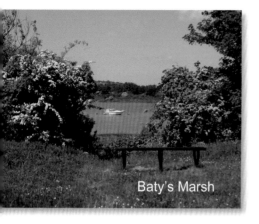

Baty's Marsh

Borstal

The first institution under a programme to separate young convicts from adults was established here in 1902 and the village gave its name to other such institutions not only in the United Kingdom but also in certain Commonwealth countries such as India.

Baty's Marsh

Formerly known as Borstal Marsh, this is a typical example of relatively uncommon fragmented saltmarsh. It is a designated Local Nature Reserve and also part of a Local Wildlife Site that includes Temple Marsh, just downstream on the opposite bank which supports rare birds such as breeding nightingales.

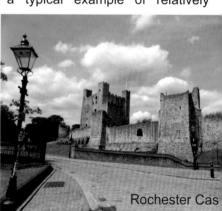

Rochester Cas

Rochester Castle

Close to the end of the walk the Water Gate, Norman in style but actually a reproduction, leads to the castle garden within the original bailey walls where there are toilets and a refreshment kiosk.

At the top of the bailey is one of the finest Norman keeps in the country, built by archbishop of Canterbury, William Corbeuil, to whom the castle passed in 1126. All the internal floors in the main body of the keep are gone but you can climb to the top and walk around the walls on two sides.

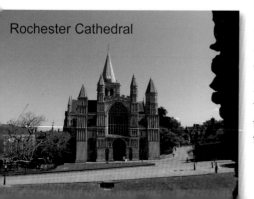

Rochester Cathedral

Rochester Cathedral

There is a fine view of the west front of the cathedral from the castle. The four turrets, the arcading and the carved doorway present a harmonious whole despite the imperfect symmetry. Three of the turrets were restored in 1892. The figures atop the inner pillars of the doorway have been variously identified as Henry I and Queen Matilda or as Solomon and the Queen of Sheba. Much of the rest of the cathedral has been rebuilt and restored over the centuries to such an extent that a simple description of who built what and when is impossible. Some love the result and some rather loathe what they see as the lack of authenticity of the restoration. It is worth a look to decide for yourself – I found the overall ambience created by the architecture and lighting quite pleasing especially the crypt which has been converted into a welcoming exhibition space.

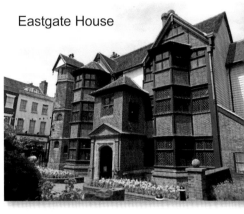
Eastgate House

Rochester High Street

In the pedestrianised High Street you will find no shortage of tea rooms, pubs and charity shops geared to the tourist market. There is a good museum in the Guildhall (free of charge, not open Mondays), a visitor information centre and a second-hand bookshop that claims to be the largest in England. Eastgate House is an Elizabethan town house that has been recently restored and reopened to the public – it was used by Charles Dickens as a model for Westgate House in *Pickwick Papers* and for The Nun's House in *Edwin Drood*.

Restoration House

On Crow Lane, just off the High Street, this red brick Elizabethan mansion was the model for *Satis House*, the home of Miss Havisham in *Great Expectations*. The name reflects Charles II's supposed stay here on his way back from France for the restoration of the monarchy. The house and garden are open to the public in summer and early autumn but not every day.

The Rochester Bridges

Rochester has long been a key crossing point on the Medway.

Restoration House

Watling Street, the Roman road from Richborough to London and beyond, crossed the river here. Soon after the 43 AD invasion, the Romans constructed nine stone piers in the river and placed a wooden walkway on top. Each of

78

the nine piers was allocated to a different group of Kent parishes, each group being responsible for the cost of repairing its allocated pier. This arrangement kept the Roman bridge in use until it was washed away by floods and ice in 1381.

The second bridge, completed in 1391, consisted of eleven arches, ten of stone and one a wooden drawbridge that could be raised to allow ships through. The drawbridge and an adjacent arch were later converted into a single stone arch, larger than the rest.

The medieval bridge was replaced in 1856 by a cast iron bridge with three arches and a swing bridge at the Strood end to allow ships upstream. The construction of railway bridges that did not allow the passage of ships made the swing bridge pointless and the whole bridge was reconstructed to its

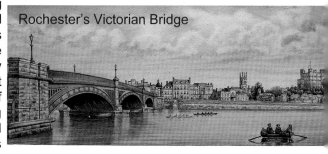

Rochester's Victorian Bridge

present form which now carries westbound traffic only. Of the two railway bridges, the one immediately downstream from the road bridge became redundant and was converted in the late 1960s to carry eastbound traffic.

The bridges are unique in being owned and maintained by a charitable trust, the Rochester Bridge Trust, which has investments and income sufficient to meet its commitments without any public funding. Hence the motto "*publica privatis*" which is liberally displayed on the westbound bridge to indicate works for the public provided by a private organisation.

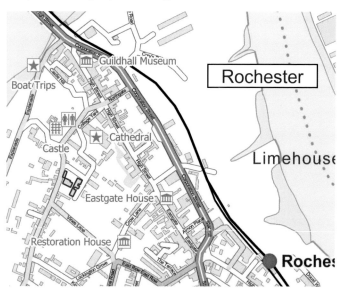

About the Ramblers

The Ramblers has been championing the interests of walkers, encouraging more people to go walking and protecting the places we walk since 1935.

We promote walking as both a pleasurable activity and as something that brings huge physical and mental health benefits to those who participate.

Our members enjoy a range of benefits, including 48,000 led walks organised by almost 500 local groups across Great Britain, access to 2,500 downloadable Ramblers Routes and our quarterly magazine, *Walk*. All walkers, from those who tackle challenging long distance trails to dog walkers exploring their local neighbourhood, benefit from the work we do.

The England Coast Path, for example, was possible because of the vision, campaigning skills and hard work of Ramblers' staff and volunteers.

The right to roam across open mountain, moorland and similar terrain also came about because of persistent campaigning by the Ramblers.

Every day our volunteers scrutinise proposals from landowners and others to close or alter public rights of way to ensure that any changes do not disadvantage walkers.

All across the country teams of volunteers are seeking to identify and claim rights of way missed off the definitive maps in the 1950s and 1960s to prevent them being extinguished in 2026 under legislation introduced in 2000.

And our local path maintenance teams clear overgrown paths and install stiles, gates and steps to help keep paths accessible and enable people to go walking in the places that they love.

Even this book represents hundreds of hours of work by Ramblers' volunteers.

There are so many reasons to join the Ramblers and help us to continue to create a Britain where everyone has the freedom to enjoy the outdoors on foot and benefit from the experience. Find out more about what you can do to support the Ramblers today at www.ramblers.org.uk.

Kent Ramblers' Volunteer
Recruitment Leaflet

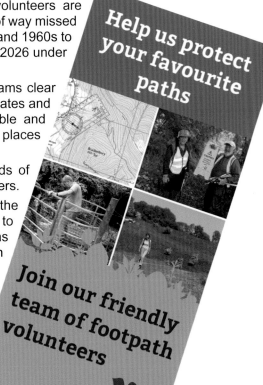

Help us protect your favourite paths

Join our friendly team of footpath volunteers

ramblers
at the heart of walking

80

Acknowledgements

Mapping

Contains OS data © Crown copyright and database rights (2018).

The base mapping is derived from Ordnance Survey data released into the public domain under the Open Government Licence.

The footpaths in Kent, Surrey and Medway are derived from data released by the respective county councils under the Open Government licence. These datasets contain data derived in part from Ordnance Survey data © Crown Copyright and database rights 2018

The national and regional cycle networks are reproduced by kind permission of Sustrans.

The routes of the three walks are based on GPS tracks made by the author.

All other information on the maps has been created by the author.

Photographs and Other Illustrations

Samuel Palmer's "In a Shoreham Garden" and Wenceslas Hollar's print of Starborough Castle: Wikimedia Commons

The photograph of Hever Castle is reproduced by kind permission of Hever Castle & Gardens. The photograph of Penshurst Place is reproduced by kind permission of Penshurst Place. The photographs of St John's Jerusalem Garden are reproduced by kind permission of the National Trust. The photograph of Allington Castle is reproduced by kind permission of the owners. The print of Rochester's Victorian bridge is reproduced by kind permission of the Rochester Bridge Trust. Photograph of hop stringing by T Edmondson.

All photographs and illustrations neither mentioned above nor specifically attributed where they appear are the work of the author.

Many thanks to those members of Kent Ramblers who have helped check this guide. Any remaining errors are, of course, those of the author.

Guide to Kent Coast Path

You may also be interested in our previous walking guide which describes the route of the first section of the England Coast Path to open in Kent. The route, running from Camber to Ramsgate, opened in 2016 and offers a varied journey past golden sands, internationally important shingle habitats, the famous white cliffs, castles of various ages, a nuclear power station and numerous other points of interest. The guide can be obtained from good bookshops both online and on the ground, or from our website: www.kentramblers.org.uk/books.

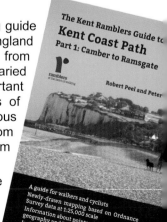

The list price is £7.50 but discounts are often to be found.